Contents

Preface   iv
Foreword   vii
About the author, Acknowledgements   viii

Section I   Spiritual need and spiritual care   1

Chapter 1   The nature of spiritual need   2
Chapter 2   The approach to spiritual care – journeying together   8

Section II   The carers   17

Chapter 3   The carer as a resource – knowing ourselves   18
Chapter 4   The carer's response to spiritual need – a relationship of equals 24
Chapter 5   The carer's skills – looking, listening and communicating   31
Chapter 6   The carer's assessment skills – putting it all together   37
Chapter 7   The carer's resources – sharing the load   45

Section III   The patient's response   53

Chapter 8   The emotional response to being a patient   54
Chapter 9   The patient's response to suffering, pain and loss   59
Chapter 10   Responding to particular aspects of suffering – why me?   68
Chapter 11   The patient's response to healing and recovery – new perspectives 81

Section IV   Provisions for meeting special needs in particular situations 89

Chapter 12   Provision for meeting particular spiritual needs –
               unexpected situations and general principles   91
Chapter 13   Provision for spiritual needs – long-term situations   102
Chapter 14   Meeting spiritual needs in different denominations or faiths   115
Chapter 15   Special needs in controversial situations, dilemmas and decisions 123

Section V   Practical issues in management and delivery of spiritual care 133

Chapter 16   The caring team – roles, relationships and responsibilities   134
Chapter 17   Resources for spiritual care – finding and facilitating   139
Chapter 18   Caring for the carers – staff have needs too   145

Section VI   Wholeness and healing in spiritual care   153

Chapter 19   Bringing it all together – the healing relationship   154

Appendix – Useful addresses and resources   158
Further reading   161
References   162
Index   166

Preface

We shall not cease from exploration
And the end of all our exploring
Will be to arrive where we started
And know the place for the first time.

TS Elliot – *Little Gidding*

Two frustrations have led to this book being written. The first lies in the confusion that is continually evident over the concepts of spiritual need and care. It exists because these terms are so often assumed to be the same as religious care and are depicted as such. Many people in the caring professions speak and write as if the words 'spiritual' and 'religious' are interchangeable.

The second frustration comes from the view, often encountered, that spiritual care is an optional extra which, if ignored, will have little impact on the patient and family. The contention that I have tried to express throughout the book is that spiritual care is essential for the well-being of everyone and is a significant factor in the care of patients, families and staff. The book has been written so that each Chapter stands on its own as well as contributing to a growing picture of the depth and complexity of spiritual need and spiritual care. It may therefore be used with or without the exercises and questions incorporated into the text.

To respond to spiritual need is demanding, but also very rewarding and creates a deep rapport between the people concerned. The book is written in the hope that all health-care professionals and voluntary carers will see the important role that each can play in valuing each and every sufferer and in easing the 'dis-ease' which suffering brings.

THE BASIC APPROACH

Spiritual care was, until recent years considered to be mainly the responsibility of the hospital chaplain or a minister of religion, priest or religious leader and requests for help were usually referred to the appropriate person for attention, and the matter was then thankfully left in their hands. Any difficult or embarrassing situations such as terminal illness, death or sudden deprivation of any kind were passed on to the 'expert' with a quiet sigh of relief.

Things are now changing radically, however, and there is currently a surge of interest in caring for the whole person and looking after their physical, emotional, social and spiritual needs. It is only too evident that many professionals are realising their need for guidance and help in playing their part in providing spiritual care. A literature review of recently published papers included articles from chaplains, nurses, psychologists and psychiatrists, doctors, counsellors, and occupational therapists, all demonstrating a high level of commitment and interest. Some of these address specific issues or deal with the needs of different groups such as the terminally ill, the bereaved, children, people needing rehabilitation or counselling, and the mentally handicapped or mentally ill. (There are references to these in the text and they are also listed at the end of the book.)

SPIRITUAL ASPECTS OF HEALTH CARE

Reverend David J Stoter AKC JP

Manager of Chaplaincy Department
and Bereavement Centre,
Queen's Medical Centre,
University Hospital Nottingham (NHS) Trust.
Chairman of the Council,
National Association for Staff Support
(for staff in the health care services).

Foreword by
Christine Hancock BSC (ECON) RGN

General Secretary,
Royal College of Nursing of the United Kingdom,
London.

M Mosby

London Baltimore Bogotá Boston Buenos Aires Caracas Carlsbad, CA Chicago Madrid Mexico City Milan Naples, FL
New York Philadelphia St. Louis Sydney Tokyo Toronto Wiesbaden

AUTHOR'S DEDICATION:

I dedicate this book with gratitude to my wife, Moira,
and my children, Mark and Claire.

Project Manager:	Louise Crowe
Publisher:	Griselda Campbell
Editorial Consultant:	Nancy Loffler
Production:	Joe Lynch
DTP Layout:	Chris Read
Template Design:	Judith Gauge
Cover Design:	Lara Last
Index:	Grace Owen

Copyright © 1995 Times Mirror International Publishers Limited

Published in 1995 by Mosby, an imprint of Times Mirror International Publishers Limited

Printed by J W Arrowsmith Ltd

ISBN 0 7234 1955 8

For full details of all Times Mirror International Publishers Limited titles, please write to Times Mirror International Publishers Limited, Lynton House, 7–12 Tavistock Square, London WC1H 9LB, UK.

A CIP catalogue record for this book is available from the British Library.

Spiritual care then is becoming a major concern for a range of professional carers who recognise the relevance of spiritual well-being in the process of recovery and its importance for those in the terminal stages of illness as it contributes to their quality of life.

THE NATURE OF THE SUBJECT

It follows that a book of this kind has to serve a wide range of needs and interests, hence the importance of understanding the basic premises on which it is based at an early stage, to get the best out of the experience of reading it.

Spiritual care is a very wide subject to approach in one book. With a growing interest in many topical issues, it would be easy to over emphasise these at the expense of other equally important but less well-documented areas. The book is therefore structured to look first at basic principles and then move on to cover general and specific areas of interest without including material likely to be out of date very quickly. The references to journal articles will enable the reader to consult these for current material. The book demonstrates the breadth of the subject through the range of aspects covered and as suggested earlier, the reader may either approach it with a view to getting a general overall perspective, or take specific Sections to study in greater depth.

THE LAYOUT OF THE BOOK

The book is divided into Sections and the Chapters within these Sections deal with various topics under their headings in a logical sequence so that the reader can proceed right through the book with each Chapter building on the ground covered in the previous one. For the serious reader who would like to use it as a reference book, each Section can also be regarded as a subject in its own right and can be read as such.

For students who wish to use the text while following a prescribed course, the book is well referenced with articles substantiating the text or giving more detailed research findings where they exist. Students may refer to the original work for more specific detail. Books are listed for further reading. At the end of each Section there are a few questions which can be used as a basis for essay topics in preparation for examination or professional qualification. The exercises suggested are designed to follow in sequence building on previous work and reflecting on any learning experiences. It would be useful to keep all the work done in a loose leaf file to be used as a record of personal study for revision or reference. The experienced practitioner may also find this book a useful resource guide.

PROGRESSION THROUGH THE BOOK

The book is written with a wide range of needs in mind, and also different levels of skill. This is a useful approach in the light of the growing surge of interest in so many areas and also with the recognition that spirituality is an integrating life force and spiritual care is everyone's concern. The opening Section seeks to clarify some of the misconceptions and difficulties associated with the nature of spiritual need and spiritual care and to distinguish it from religious care.

Section II begins with the carers and their needs as it is important to first establish the fundamental basis from which the various aspects of spiritual care are approached. The skills, understanding, attitudes and experience of the carer are vital ingredients, as are the resources to back them up, in assessing need and offering spiritual care.

Section III explores some responses of individual sufferers, looking at the place of models in planning and offering care and bringing this dimension into focus to promote total care. It examines the responses to a range of different aspects of suffering. It also considers the family and other carers and friends.

In this context, Section IV goes on to explore in detail the practical aspects of meeting these needs for different individuals, groups and in specific situations in the light of social, cultural and religious backgrounds and influences. It gives useful practical guidance on meeting these specific needs covering a wider sphere of influence in special areas of care and looks at some controversial ethical issues relating to health care.

The following Section looks at practical issues such as how to locate and use resources, who to go to for help, and how and where to get further training and preparation for this aspect of care and support. Finally, it seeks to explore spiritual care in terms of its integrating function and contribution in establishing spiritual well being and finding meaning and purpose in the process of recovery.

Each reader may find the book has different uses at different stages of his or her development and practice and, if it is used in the appropriate way, it is hoped it will enable individuals and groups to move forward in their own exploration of how to walk alongside those in need of spiritual care. It may be helpful to use the book as a general reader or as an introduction to new areas of responsibility. In addition it may be useful to come back to some Chapters after a period of consolidation following some practical experience. It can also be used as an individual study book, as a basis for a course, or for group activities.

David J Stoter
Nottingham 1995

Foreword

The issue of what constitutes spiritual care has been the subject of intense debate in recent years. Politicians have scolded the Church for intervening in political matters while neglecting what they perceive to be the real spiritual needs of the nation. Meanwhile, both seem to believe that there is currently a spiritual malaise in society.

Clearly, spirituality is not as simple as some would have us believe. It cannot be compartmentalised. As *Spiritual Aspects of Health Care* shows, spirituality is about more than just religious belief. It touches upon and influences every sphere of our lives. That is why in health care there has been a growing awareness of the importance of spiritual support alongside the physical and emotional aspects of care. There has been a far greater emphasis on providing holistic care, treating the whole person and not just the condition. Indeed, with the prevalence of stress related conditions and mental illness in society, treatment and health promotion activity will increasingly require an understanding of the spiritual dimension in peoples' lives, even if that dimension is not immediately obvious.

The development of new medical technology, for example keyhole and minimally invasive surgery, has inevitably raised peoples' expectations of the care they receive. However, even if technology may save their lives, many people will have to come to terms with living with an altered body shape. They may need help with performing basic functions for the rest of their lives. At the same time, there will always be those who refuse invasive surgery, no matter how minimal. These patients may require greater pain management or palliative care; they will almost certainly have spiritual needs of which they themselves may not be aware.

For people involved in accidents or catastrophes, and their families and friends, bereavement and trauma counselling is assuming more and more importance in their overall care. Spiritual care is an important element of this process. In some cases, it could be the only effective care available.

Spiritual Aspects of Health Care addresses spiritual care from every perspective: the needs of carers as well as patients. It shows how carers can acquire the skills and resources to provide the right sort of care, and how they can establish a healing relationship in which to explore the spiritual dimension.

The book is also an important resource in terms of staff support. Its highly accessible, practical approach to the issues surrounding spiritual support make it an invaluable tool for all health care professionals in caring for others and understanding their own spiritual needs in the care environment.

Christine Hancock
General Secretary
Royal College of Nursing of the United Kingdom

About the author

David Stoter started his training as a Priest at King's College, London, and completed it at Warminster Theological College. After an initial period as a Curate, he took up his first hospital appointment as Chaplain of Luton and Dunstable Hospital in 1970, subsequently moving to Westminster Hospital for seven years. In 1979 he became Chaplain of the General Hospital in Nottingham and when services were transferred to Queen's Medical Centre, Nottingham, he and his team moved to this location.

Queen's Medical Centre is one of the largest teaching hospitals in Europe with the busiest Accident and Emergency Department in the United Kingdom. It encompasses all aspects of the human condition from birth, to major illness and death. David Stoter has dedicated his professional life to spiritual care in a difficult and demanding environment for the Church, and this book bears testimony to his knowledge and wisdom in providing spiritual support to those in greatest need and at the time of greatest life crisis. The demands made on staff working under these circumstances must not be overlooked and there is an excellent section of guidance for the support of staff who are often themselves deeply affected by the tragedies that they may share on a day-to-day basis. There are numerous examples to illustrate the difficulties of communication where grief and anger often combine. Medical and nursing staff sometimes find great difficulty in knowing how to respond to these situations and it is to be hoped that this book will find its way to bookshelves of all grades of staff committed to caring for the sick and the dying.

Professor E M Symonds
Dean of the Faculty of Medicine and Health Sciences
and Professor of Obstetrics
Dean of the Medical School
Queen's Medical Centre, Nottingham

Acknowledgements

My thanks are due and given warmly to a number of people who have assisted in the preparation of this book:

To Grace Owen FRCN, for interpreting my tapes and written scribbles, and also for her comments and suggestions during the writing of the book. My thanks also for her painstaking work in researching the references and indexing the text.

Also to Janet Morriss for help with typing and presentation, to Barbara Davies for putting the main text onto disk for the publishers and to Heather Bond for help with proofreading. Finally, my thanks to Nancy Loffler for her patience in negotiating this book through to the publication stage.

Section 1

Spiritual need and spiritual care

These opening Chapters outline some of the current thinking on the nature of spirituality. From here it is possible to look at definitions of 'spiritual need' and 'spiritual care'. Chapter 2 broadens upon these to look at the nature of the relationships fundamental to spiritual care and the concepts of a partnership between patient and carer in journeying together. It touches briefly on the various issues involved, laying the foundations for the following Chapters to explore the various aspects of spiritual care in detail. To complete the picture these are brought together in the last Chapter.

The nature of spiritual need

We had the experience but missed the meaning,
And approach to the meaning restores the experience
In a different form, beyond any meaning
We can assign to happiness, I have said before
That the past experience revived in the meaning
Is not the experience of one life only
But of many generations....

TS Elliot – *The Dry Salvages*

Those who are seriously concerned with caring for individuals, either in sickness or in health, are likely to be familiar with the holistic approach to care. This recognises the importance of considering the physical, social, emotional and spiritual aspects of need and care. Much attention is given to the first three of these but the spiritual dimension is too often overlooked or dismissed as an aspect of care 'best left to the clergy or to the religious leader'. This omission is probably caused by spirituality often being ill defined, misunderstood, and surrounded by misconceptions and unanswered questions. It will make our explorations easier if before we look at the nature of spiritual care, we address what is understood by the word 'spiritual' in this context.

People involved with the day-to-day care of the sick are not alone in finding the concept of spirituality difficult. Until recently, very few writers on this subject attempted to define the spiritual dimension of personality, particularly in relation to the field of health or medical care (Owen *et al.*, 1989). Members of an international conference of experts held at Yale University in 1986 faced a bewildering range of difficulties when they addressed this issue in relation to hospice care (Wald, 1986; Kreidler, 1978)

EXERCISE 1
Before reading further, it is a useful exercise to discuss and perhaps write down your present understanding of the meanings of the terms 'spiritual' and 'spirituality'. Put these aside, then at the end of the Chapter look at your definitions and add anything new you have learned.

THE SPIRITUAL COMPONENT OF NEED AND CARE

To see spiritual care only as religious care limits and diminishes its true nature and tends to relegate it to a footnote at the end of the ward report, or something to be handed on to another professional. The first step then is to distinguish between the meanings of 'spiritual' and 'religious' and to dismiss some of the confusion. The concept of 'spirituality' has traditional associations with religion. Even the Oxford dictionary tends to perpetuate the religious connotations attached to its definitions! The first definition given, however, describes 'spiritual' as 'pertaining to the spirit of Man' and 'spirit' is elsewhere defined as the 'vital principle of Man' or as the 'breath of life which gives life to the physical organism'.

Maybe this gives us an important starting point indicating, as it does, that the spiritual nature of Man is the total personality which links aspects together, and is expressed through relationships, personal practices and beliefs (Laburn, 1988). The spiritual dimension has also been described as a 'unifying force that integrates and transcends the physical, emotional and social dimensions'. It enables the search for meaning in life and provides a common bond between individuals – an essential ingredient for any relationship (Socken and Carson, 1987).

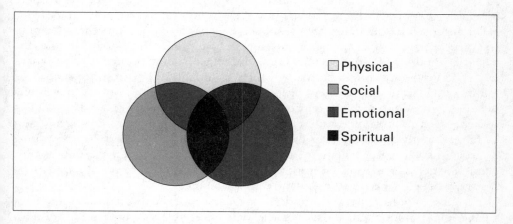

□ Physical
■ Social
■ Emotional
■ Spiritual

The nature of the SPIRITUAL DIMENSION.

Every person is a spiritual being having a spiritual dimension and thus spiritual need is universal. Spirituality may or may not include religious rituals and behaviours (Reed, 1987), and not everyone has a religious dimension. A person without a faith, however, does have a spiritual dimension and so everyone has spiritual needs. Spirituality encompasses the whole range of a person's life experiences and is influenced by these experiences. Hence, the nature of spirituality and the way in which it is expressed will vary with a person's background and culture and in the context of the framework of his particular beliefs. So the expression of need is unique to each individual.

The religious aspect of spiritual care is just one important component of spirituality and is related to the beliefs, preferences and practices of each person. Spiritual need is sometimes recognised, felt and expressed by the individual and sometimes it is not. Not everything essential to a patient's recovery is recognised as a need by the patient in terms of physical care, and similarly patients do not always recognise and express their spiritual needs.

The whole range of a person's life experiences influences the nature and uniqueness of that person's spirituality, shaping a unique capacity to respond to all life's events and situations. There are influences relating to place of birth in terms of the home conditions and quality of life in that place. To be born in a famine stricken area of Ethiopia is vastly different from being born in an affluent country. The geographical place of birth is likely to influence a person's religious affiliation and practices which, as already discussed, is a distinct component of their spirituality. The nature of an individual's family background, cultural environment, wealth and social class all have their own contributions to the development of personality. There are significant environmental influences, particularly in terms of education, work experience and security or insecurity related to affluence and wealth. These generate individual values such as self-esteem, ideals concerning achievement, failure and success, values relating to work and loss of job, and responses to other experiences through which a person lives.

There are also the influences of family and other wider relationships which affect a person's emotional development, influencing their ability to enter into other relationships. Bonding in the early years is a particularly important event in forming the capacity to love, trust and communicate effectively with others. As life unfolds for each person there is a unique and cumulative effect from the range of experiences entered into – some good and happy, others traumatic and distressing. Success or failure in marriage, bereavement or loss of any kind, and happy or unhappy family life are all experiences which contribute to an individual's perspective on life and his or her responses to people and events. The nature of support given during a period of bereavement or trauma can influence receptivity and the way in which they approach adversity. For many of the older generation, influences such as war, economic depression, social deprivation and other historical or social happenings may have deep effects on attitudes and outlook on life.

For most people, experience in their particular journey through life influences what is important to them and at one level helps to establish their personal attitudes to life, death and loss. It may affect the nature of their personality and the things they enjoy such as walking in the countryside, or the need to be a 'workaholic.' It will affect their expectations of life in a powerful way – for example, parents can have a lasting influence on the self-image of a child striving to reflect the image of the person projected onto them and this can create problems for self-esteem in later life.

'Understanding human needs is half the job of meeting them'
Adam Stevenson

EXERCISE 2
Do the same as in Exercise 1 – discuss and enter your own definitions of spiritual needs and save them to review at the end of the Chapter.

❊

THE NATURE OF SPIRITUAL NEED

Before looking at the nature of spiritual need, it is important to establish that the concept of need is in itself identified and understood. Many people talk about 'need' when they are really concerned with 'wants' and this further complicates an already complex issue. There are a few theoretical definitions available which may be helpful in this particular context. One of the models most frequently applied to health care and related issues lies within Maslow's hierarchy of human needs which embraces physiological needs, needs of safety, love and belonging, self-esteem, recognition and self-actualization (Maslow, 1954). Most carers are familiar with these aspects and this could be a useful model for understanding spiritual need because, in application, it allows for the patient or client to set personal goals on a level which can be achieved within his or her potential capacity, rather than attempting to reach goals set by someone else.

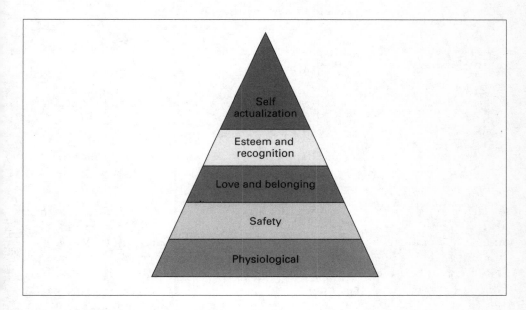

Maslow's hierarchy of needs (Maslow, 1954).

Another helpful approach is found in Bradshaw's *Taxonomy of Human Need* (1972). He bases his classification on criteria for recognition of need. He uses four definitions: normative, felt, expressed and comparative needs. A normative definition of needs is set by professional carers, and individuals who fall short of having such needs met are defined as 'in need'. This approach is open to value judgments. An approach that is currently more acceptable involves 'consumer participation' and includes 'felt need' which may of course be similar to 'wants' – therefore felt need alone is an inadequate indicator to aid our understanding.

Expressed need is often most easily identifiable as it is apparent in the formation of self-help groups or 'demand from the consumer'. Comparative need is more complex again as it involves various aspects of equity and relative equality. This approach has many implications for the carer who needs knowledge and understanding of the person's past experiences and background to understand the intensity of their need. It is involved in any decision to standardise provision (*see Chapter 13–15 for examples*). There are aspects of each of these criteria, however, which provide food for thought for the carer. Bradshaw uses an integrated model combining all four of these. This may help the carer to clarify his or her own approach to a realistic recognition of 'need', particularly in the context of spiritual care. We shall be showing the importance of understanding these definitions as more practical aspects of spiritual need are identified later in this book.

EXERCISE 3

This outline of Bradshaw's taxonomy may be used as a guide for you to work out some examples of your own from time to time as you read on through the text:

Normative needs—The expert or professional sets previously agreed standards which can be compared with existing standards in a particular situation. Where these are not met the individual is assessed as being in need.

Felt needs—These needs are limited by the individual's own perceptions where they have a desire for a service they may not need.

Expressed needs—When felt needs that have been experienced are turned into action and may reflect what is available.

Comparative needs—These relate to a person who is not receiving certain services when others in similar situations get help.

That spiritual need is universal does not necessarily mean every individual recognises their own need. This indicates the importance for carers to show sensitivity in recognising whether they are dealing with something that is not always openly acknowledged but is nevertheless present only not expressed. When this unspoken need is handled sensitively, the help offered may be received and can then contribute towards recovery. The basic spiritual help each person needs is to be seen, recognised, known and valued for itself, although this may not always be acknowledged in these terms.

When someone is grappling internally with what is happening to them, they do so in the light of the knowledge, experiences and patterns of response built up over the years. Particular values, principles, fears and aspirations are an integral part of personality. Each individual's real need is to be accepted just for themselves and to receive a response that makes them feel at peace and comfortable within themselves. This may include the need to help unravel threatening areas of pain and difficulty so facilitating the search for peace. Accepting a person's spirituality may also involve accepting a whole range of emotions the sufferer is experiencing, empathising with all the confusion and conflict through which they are passing. Their real need is to find some kind of meaning and purpose in their situation and to discover a way forward, moving towards a physical or mental recovery, or indeed moving towards death or the acceptance of loss or chronic illness.

Part of that spiritual need is to be heard as a person who has particular family or personal relationships and who is part of a particular cultural environment with particular beliefs, creed or code. The need is to be heard as somebody respected and valued. This is vitally important when coming to terms with possible loss of some of the familiar aspects of living.

EXERCISE 4
Now go back to Exercises 1 and 2 and decide how you can change and improve on your own definitions – what is new and what is puzzling for you? Keep your conclusions to re-discuss them later in the book.

❋

Spiritual needs differ considerably from one person to another, and so people find expression and satisfaction of those needs in different ways. This may be through the sacraments or corporate worship within their own faith. Maybe they do not feel it necessary or even possible to join in any corporate activity and would be happier with personal ministry, simply companionship and a listening ear, opportunities for reflection, music or meditation, or no specific provision.

In this Chapter, we have sought to distinguish between the nature of spiritual need and religious need as a basis for exploring spiritual care. Whatever the need, it is important for carers to understand the true nature of the concept of spirituality and to make the widest kind of provision for addressing individual preferences and needs.

Key points

- Holistic care includes responding to physical, social, emotional and spiritual need.
- The first three of these receive much attention but the spiritual dimension is often overlooked or misunderstood.
- It is important to define spiritual need and to distinguish it from religious need.
- Spiritual need is universal in the human race.
- Spiritual need is influenced by the whole range of life's experiences, cultural and personal.
- These experiences are unique to each individual, so spiritual needs will differ accordingly.

CHAPTER

2

The approach to spiritual care: journeying together

But the prolonged journey was necessary since it is only the truth that you discover for yourself which has the power of truth. To be told something is seldom to know it, however numerous the instructors ... further, the more earnest they are, the less convincing.

Harry Williams – *Some Day I'll Find You*

EXERCISE 5

Before you embark on this Chapter repeat Exercises 1 and 2, this time using the definitions of 'spiritual care' and 'religious care' as you have practised them in your own professional role.

In the context of spiritual need, as defined in the previous Chapter, spiritual care can be described as responding to the uniqueness of the individual: accepting their range of doubts, beliefs and values just as they are. It means responding to the spoken or unspoken statements from the very core of that person as valid expressions of where they are and who they are. It is to be a facilitator in their search for identity on the journey of life and in the particular situation in which they find themselves. It is to respond without being prescriptive, judgmental or dogmatic and without preconditions, acknowledging that each will be at a different stage on that personal spiritual journey.

For spiritual care to be effective, the carer has first to identify the need or needs that are present by listening to and accepting each person as and where they are. Second, in order to be able to offer spiritual care at all, the carer must be acceptable to the person receiving the care. In general terms, spiritual care can be offered through an attitude of love and acceptance within the caring relationship.

However, moving into deeper levels needs a caring relationship or contract to be firmly established where the recipient can accept the carer as someone who can be entrusted with all their needs, hopes and fears, pains and distresses and to whom they can entrust themselves fully and totally. They are able to trust in that way because they recognise their needs will be received and handled sensitively and that the carer has something to offer. The focus of the care must be for the good of the patient or client, without preconditions or any specific end in view, and without particular objectives forcing the individual into a particular place or response to satisfy the carer. Spiritual care then is a 'gift of love offered with no preconditions' (Stoter, 1991). ✳

Trungpa (1978) writes:

> .... the healing relationship is a meeting of two minds: the healer
> and the patient ... If you and the other person are both open, then
> some kind of dialogue can take place .... communication occurs
> naturally. From the patient's point of view that is exactly what is
> needed!
>
> Trung Pa – *Acknowledging Death*

Spiritual care, as all care, needs to be centred around the patient and, to that end, it is always the client's perspectives, desires and objectives which are of highest priority and importance and not those of the carers. This is an equation which is frequently reversed in order to reinforce the worth and self-esteem of the carer. The core of spiritual care is to value each individual for themselves, to accept them just where they are with their own particular needs and attitudes. One acceptable objective is to enable the individual to accept and value themselves and to make some meaning of whatever situation they are in, and to discover their own way forward on life's journey in a way which is acceptable and creative for them.

Preaching, proselytising and coercion, or any form of moral or religious blackmail are all unacceptable in this context and completely unhelpful. These issues will all be explored more fully at a later stage in this book. The positive response to this aspect of meeting spiritual needs was well summarised in a statement offered at a previously mentioned conference at Yale University – 'it should be the patient who defines the territory, not the caregiver' (Fiefel, 1986).

DEFINING THE TERRITORY

> *Is not religion all deeds and all reflection,*
> *And that which is neither deed nor reflection*
> *but a wonder and surprise ever springing in the soul,*
> *even while hands hew the stone or tend the loom?*
> *Who can separate his faith from his actions,*
> *or his belief from his occupations?*
>
> Kahlil Gibran – *The Prophet*

Religious care

Religious care is just one aspect or one component of spiritual care which attempts to meet spiritual needs, recognising the influences that make a person the kind of individual that they are. Religion has been aptly described as 'the arena of faith in practice, such as affiliation with a particular church or synagogue', or activities practised within a specific faith (Bowers, 1987). We are all born into a particular spiritual culture, aspects of which clearly influence our attitudes, thinking and personality. As we have already mentioned, spirituality is universal and is more appropriately related to the realm of human needs, which may find expression within particular religious practices.

It is important to emphasise the significance of learning in the earliest years of life – learning which takes place without analysis or understanding. We take on board in those early years our environmental culture as the norm of life as we know no alternative then. At the same time, the powerful cultural, spiritual and religious attitudes of our parents and surrounding family are absorbed at a very deep level and without question or analysis. This can influence markedly our responses in later life and our ways of coping with life. Sometimes very heavy influences from dogmatic parents are so powerful and dominant that they can influence or inhibit thinking and relationships throughout life unless the position is reached where there is a positive recognition of these influences and an attempt to come to terms with their effects. Such influences can also by their nature create an 'anti-response' because of the parents' strong attitudes and the environment in which they are established. This all has a very strong bearing on a person's religious affiliation and preferences.

Religious care is care given by members of a specific faith or religious community. Frequently, it is given by appointed leaders to bring resources and practices of that particular faith and group alongside the individual who is in need. This can be done in many different ways. During the course of this book we will be looking at some of the helpful and unhelpful practices and responses which may be brought to the bedside or presented to the client. One important question to be faced in this area is whether giving religious care should be in line with a rigorous application of an already predetermined range of responses or practices which are universally applied, or whether the care given needs to be more personally designed to respond to the specific needs of the person as they are acknowledged.

One example of this would be the use of a special sacramental ministry, which could involve the administration of the sacrament or a specific use of prayer at the bedside. Another issue to consider would be whether it is more appropriate for the leader of the community or faith to 'walk with' the patient, or is it preferable for the patient to follow the one ministering to them?

The starting point for our exploration of spiritual care is to recognise that everyone has a spiritual dimension and that for some people the religious dimension is just one component of this universal need. Each individual has certain personal beliefs and values which together with environmental and cultural influences make him or her a unique person. Spiritual need will therefore vary from one individual to another. Needs are expressed differently and are relative to other conditions and so may change from time to time. It is not then possible to make sweeping assumptions about the needs of people as there are no set answers. This is probably why the subject is so often avoided and felt to be threatening, as the perceived issues are very complex ones.

When offering spiritual care it is important to recognise this universal need for acceptance and affirmation and also the need to help the individual to discover the way forward in a caring and understanding environment. Cicely Saunders refers to the natural inclination of care givers to decide what is best for the patient before fully understanding what the patient wants for him or herself. The patient sets the goals and the carer helps him to use his personal resources '....the patient should be in the centre. The question is his because it is his situation and he is the person who matters' (Saunders, 1969). This approach is central to the philosophy of this book and also to the provision of spiritual care, which must be considered as having an integral contribution towards the delivery of total care for the whole person.

THE SPIRITUAL JOURNEY

The nature of spiritual need and spiritual care as described in the first chapter clearly indicates that the carer's approach has to be through coming alongside the patient or client and sharing the journey of life at whatever point that person finds himself at that particular time.

The spiritual journey

When we prepare to go on a journey of any kind, in the normal course of events, we are faced with a range of different ways of travelling or journeying. In some situations, a definite programme is offered and, if attracted by this programme, one may choose to join in. For example, this may mean joining a group for a planned ramble or excursion following a particular route to a known destination. It may mean going on a holiday with an advertised schedule, a planned daily itinerary. This is clearly an official programme and, as such, is known and accepted when one joins a journey of that kind. It is possible, however, for the participant to relate more positively to some aspects of the programme than others that have a lesser appeal.

Then there are less formal kinds of journeys, such as when someone says, 'I am going on a journey to...., would you like to come with me?' Here there is a choice of whether the individual wants to go to that place with that person. Alternatively, you may get an open invitation to spend a day with someone where no set plan is indicated beforehand. Yet another example is found when two people get together and say, 'Let's share a walk together and enjoy the country'. This entails a mutual agreement on where to go.

However, on the journey we are considering here – the journey of life – the patient or client is already on their particular path. The situation they find themselves in may mean they are facing particular challenges, questions and decisions. They have no choice about where they are, where they start from or the final destination ahead. The carer, on the other hand, has a great deal of power: power to choose whether to share that journey at all; power to decide how far to go and when to pull out; and power to leave the path altogether if so wished. The carer also has the ability to put parameters in place or to define the territory. This makes it impossible for the recipient to follow his own personal journey, as it suggests that either the carer 'knows best what is right' and where the traveller should go, or is going to insist on controlling every aspect of the journey.

It is also important for many travellers to be able to recognise the itinerary, to know what the journey entails and its anticipated destination, and so be able to consciously plan their route, finding a sense of security and fulfilment so that their particular needs, hopes and aims are being realised.

Journeying together

Campbell (1984) suggests that companionship on this journey arises from a chance meeting where the two individuals 'come together by chance'. The joint purpose in such a relationship is moving onward either to recovery or to death (Bayntun-Lees, 1992). This involves many issues relating to the 'partnership' between patient and carer, which will be fully explored in Chapter 4.

As carers attempting to travel with a patient, client or relative, it is important to recognise our own vulnerability and limitations and to identify areas where we ourselves feel threatened, particularly where the territory is unfamiliar or unfriendly, or lies outside our own experience. The carer retains the power to keep within the territory or to establish the parameters of safety for himself. The danger arises when this does not coincide with the patient's own perception of his journey and the carer is prevented from coming alongside.

True companionship is established on the spiritual journey just as in any other journey when two people walk together, see the same scenery and respond to their environment and to one another at different levels and in different dimensions. On the surface they share their responses to the experiences of the walk and what they see around them, but there are deeper perspectives to be observed. Each can help the other to recognise what has never been noticed before as they walk through the territory together sharing the responses and emotions it evokes.

As they enter into this deeper level of sharing together, the travellers may find themselves moving nearer together – not simply physically but coming closer at a deeper personal level in mind, heart and spirit. Sometimes on this kind of journey where experiences are shared, it may happen that the travellers find they are not going to reach the original destination as anticipated, but they are able to value the unexpected discoveries made *en route*. There may be the bonus of finding a hitherto unknown oasis in the desert, giving a temporary resting place with time for refreshment and to revise plans. Alternatively, when the everyday pressures of life are removed, the more leisurely journey may allow time to step aside and discover a previously unnoticed viewpoint that reveals new horizons and enables adjustments to be made to the route travelled. Such opportunities bring many compensations, which may be missed on a more rigid schedule, and which help to make up for other disappointments encountered.

For those of us who are carers, starting where the other person is means to be willing to stand aside from our own journey and to allow the agenda and itinerary to be set by the patient or client. It may well be something of a mystery tour, complicated by the starting points and itinerary needing to be discovered afresh at each meeting. When we leave a person for a while and return later to resume a relationship, we can never expect to meet at the same place as we left off. Both of us will have met with fresh experiences and insights, seen new horizons and have moved into a new phase of the journey or quickened the pace in the intervening time. We need to get in step with each other once more as we move along and share in the next stage of the journey.

EXERCISE 6
This exercise is probably best carried out personally, as people's experiences will vary:
- Sketch out in brief what you see as your own 'spiritual journey' noting the route by which you have travelled and some of the turning points for you. Ideally it helps to clarify where you think you are at present and to check this from time to time as you read on. It can be a progressive exercise.
- Set out some of the beliefs and values that indicate where you stand at present. What were the major influences shaping these beliefs and values.

> *Fare forward travellers! not escaping from the past*
> *Into different lives, or into any future;*
> *You are not the same people who left that station*
> *Or who will arrive at any terminus,*
> *While the narrowing rails slide together behind you;*
> *You are not those who saw the harbour*
> *Receding, or those who will disembark.*
>
> TS Eliot – *The Dry Salvages*

SOME ISSUES TO EXPLORE WHEN JOURNEYING TOGETHER

This approach presents difficulties for some carers who find themselves threatened by the unpredictability of such a relationship. This is where carers themselves need help and support to enter into sharing a journey of this kind. Some of these aspects of spiritual care, together with the resources available for help, will be explored in more detail later on in this book looking at the implications for practice.

EXERCISE 7
You have indicated where you stand on your journey in life – now consider someone you have cared for and describe how you would discuss where they have arrived on their journey. What are some of the clues you would look for?

> *As has been said, the point of travelling is not to arrive, but to return home*
> *laden with pollen you shall work up into the honey the mind feeds on.*
>
> RS Thomas – *Somewhere*

The threat of the unknown

When people are ill, and particularly in times of very serious illness, they are to a greater or lesser extent in an alien country and uncharted territory. They often feel threatened just by being in hospital in unfamiliar surroundings and separated from family and friends. They may feel threatened by the simplest of diagnostic tests, surgery, treatment and by any new experience. These factors may raise considerable fear and anxiety in the patient at different levels. The fear may sound unreasonable: fears of needles, anaesthetics, blood, or pain, fears even of looking silly or childish, or thinking they are alone in finding things frightening and difficult to accept. They may also find it hard to trust those who care for them. They will form their own perceptions of the skills and abilities of their carers, often with very accurate assessments.

Example

An example to illustrate this is seen in the child who was receiving a bone marrow transplant and being nursed in an isolation tent to prevent infection. He amused himself by drawing lifelike pictures of the staff who cared for him. He drew all of them holding syringes of varying shapes and sizes. Some of these had enormous drops of blood around the tip of the needle and were obviously more blunt than others. These drawings were his personal assessment of the skills of the individual members of staff.

Illness also raises fears and anxieties at a deeper level: fears about the future, perhaps related to past experience. Questions arise such as: 'Will I be able to cope?'; 'Will the operation be successful, and shall I be able to do the same as before – hold my job down?'; 'Will I be able to continue to be an effective husband, wife or parent?'; 'Will I be able to do the same things as before – to run, swim, cycle, drive etc.?' All of these feelings become major issues and are very rational fears.

Fears about death

There may also be fears and thoughts about mortality, perhaps for the first time, as the possibility of not being alive for much longer is confronted. There are fears about what happens at death and beyond: 'Is there anything or anyone there?'. Painful as it may be, patients also experience fears about the family: 'What will happen if I leave them? Will they cope? Will they even miss me?' Alternatively, 'Will anyone ever miss me? Have I ever done anything useful in life, made my mark? Who am I? Who will miss me? Do I matter to anyone?'. All of these and countless other questions may arise at some time during any illness and they are part of the spiritual challenge.

Sometimes there is a tension between wanting the family to cope alone and yet at the same time feeling, 'If they do cope alone I can't mean very much to them. Who will care if I go ? Do I matter any more?'. For most people uncertainties arise about the possibility of not being able to do things which they have always done before. Some of these questions may be expressed verbally, but sometimes they are left unsaid and are only recognisable by indirect statements, by a throw-away line, a look, the droop of the body or the lifelessness of the eyes.

Example

An elderly man was admitted to hospital on the request of his GP as it was becoming impossible to care for him at home, particularly as he had suddenly become aggressive, constantly venting his anger and frustration on his family, who could no longer cope. He had previously been a mild and gentle man and no one could discover the cause of the change.

After a while in hospital he was able to open up and talk about his frustration. He had been a keen and able DIY person who cared competently for his property, and when he had become bedridden he lay in bed looking out onto his garden feeling helpless. The crunch came when one day he saw a ladder being placed outside his window and watched a plumber climbing up to do some repairs to the gutter. He knew he could no longer do the work he loved, but his anger grew as he realised he was not now consulted in these matters or told what was happening. His family had wished to spare him the worry, while he would have enjoyed being involved in the decisions made. He felt useless and left out with no part to play.

Once he had been able to talk about this, it opened up the way to review the situation with his family and to relieve some of his frustration, allowing him to be involved in family decisions again and restoring his sense of worth. He became much more peaceful and more like his former self again, and able to be cared for at home.

Questions and answers

These are some of the questions the carer needs to expect as well as being sensitive to the spoken and unspoken fears and aware of some of the internal processes as people struggle with life-and-death issues related to what is happening to them. Later in the book we shall explore in some detail how to be prepared to understand these internal processes which are going on all the time and how to respond to such questions. After all, we all ask questions at a very mundane level each day such as what to eat, what to wear, or where to go on holiday. These very basic questions often preoccupy us, so we should be prepared for basic questions related to the illness to be raised.

The difficulty for the carer is that there are no definitive answers, especially to those arising from the depths of feeling. It is in the carer's hand to help to forge a relationship in which feelings and uncertainties can be shared and expressed – particularly feelings of despair, helplessness and hopelessness, which may, at times, overwhelm the patient. It needs skill to bring these questions into the open and sensitivity to come alongside a person at that level, to meet their genuine expressions and feelings of insecurity, fear or anger with sincerity and without platitudes.

EXERCISE 8

This can be a useful discussion in a group – identify some of the questions you have been asked by patients and look at ways in which you have approached the answers.

We have many challenges to consider on different issues and this book cannot provide all the answers (often there are none). It will attempt, however, to encourage an exploration, for those of us who are carers, into our own personal spiritual nature and needs and to understand our own perspectives and prejudices more fully . It will also encourage exploration into understanding what is happening to the patient and relatives during this difficult period. It will seek to encourage a willingness to develop the necessary skills to expose ourselves to the challenge of caring for the whole person and not just to meet superficial needs. It also aims at being willing to stand aside at one level from our own spiritual journey and agenda, and to draw alongside and share the journey with the one we are caring for.

It is therefore important for the carer to establish a relationship with the patient in which the spiritual journey can be shared and not just to remain a detached observer in the distance while reading this book.

This Section has concentrated on clarifying some of the misconceptions about spiritual care, offering definitions and attempting to open up aspects of the approach to care, introducing the analogy of an exploratory journey. The two people who are most intimately concerned with this process of exploration are the patient and the carer and this leads us into the next two Sections, which concentrate on both the carer's and patient's needs and on responses within the context of this relationship.

Key points

- Definition and identification of spiritual care.
- A prerequisite for offering spiritual care is a caring relationship or contract between two people, which is client-centred.
- The territory needs to be defined – also a definition of religious care as an aspect of spiritual care.
- Everyone has a spiritual dimension and therefore spiritual need is universal.
- The nature of that need may differ between individuals – individual needs are shaped by early environmental influences.
- Individual needs vary and are unique to each person.
- The approach to spiritual care is through meeting a patient or client at a particular point in his personal spiritual journey.
- Each person journeys at a different pace and by different routes.
- The carer needs to identify where the patient is on his journey and come to travel alongside for as long as it takes.
- Some of the issues they need to share may be challenging to the carer because of personal differences.
- These differences need to be identified and will be explored in detail later.

Section II

The carers

The first area to consider in detail is the nature of the partnership referred to in the first Section. The major resources to consider are the carers (family, friends or professionals) and the patient or client. This Section concentrates on the carers, exploring in some detail the personal skills and resources they bring into the caring relationship. It also looks at the importance of being aware of the nature and the contribution they make, and how they influence the carer's response to spiritual need. This forms the core of the relationship between carer and patient. The carer's skills are considered in some detail, especially the ways in which these skills contribute towards assessment of need, and facilitate the carer's response. Finally, the section looks at these resources within the team and the way in which the resources can be used most effectively in providing total care.

CHAPTER 3

The carer as a resource – knowing ourselves

See first that you yourself deserve to be a giver,
and an instrument of giving.
For in truth it is life that gives unto life.
You give but little when you give of your possessions.
It is when you give of yourself that you truly give.

Kahlil Gibran—*The Prophet*

Anyone in a caring relationship acceptable to the person to be cared for is clearly in a relationship in which they become a resource. One of the issues we need to address when looking at spiritual care is just how wide and how deep that resourcing may become. It is clearly possible to look at a patient or family and to choose needs which can be responded to easily and simply and to address those needs with which the carer feels comfortable and in charge.

It is also possible to keep caring at a professional level at which physical needs are magnified above all others. We shall return to the issues of establishing relationships with the patient and family, to look at them in greater depth, at a later stage in this book. Here it is important for the carer to recognise areas where they already feel confident as a competent resource. This usually tends to begin at a level of responding to the obvious and identifiable physical needs which the illness or situation indicates.

Perhaps one smoke screen which can obscure the true level of care is to misinterpret acts of kindness as acts of caring, although kindness can be a significant part of that caring. Carers frequently undervalue or misunderstand the way in which they themselves are a resource and purveyor of spiritual care, consequently they look around for things to do. For the carer, whether staff or relative, this can lead to the 'fussing syndrome'; for example, perpetually tidying the bedside locker, fussing with sheets or constantly asking the patient if he would like a drink. This is often a reflection of the carer's feeling of utter helplessness, which is expressed in this way when there is nothing else that can be done or given on the physical level. Clearly there are times when this can be an irritant to the patient.

It certainly demands a depth of personal awareness and self-development and, not infrequently, a lot of courage to enable the carer to make him or herself available as a resource. It demands giving oneself and exposing one's vulnerability, allowing the interaction of two or more people in depth. Certain questions and feelings arise for the carer, such as, 'What have I to offer? What can I do to help?' and 'When looking at the situation I feel so helpless – I find it hard to enter that room, or to go to that bedside because I just don't know what to say or do.' Perhaps the more appropriate question to ask ourselves would be 'What does the patient want or need from me now?'. This would focus attention on to the patient's need rather than on what the carer wants to offer.

THE CARER'S PERSONAL RESOURCES – EARLY INFLUENCES

What then are the resources the carer can bring to these situations? It is most important to remember that each person has laid down a unique resource of experience and knowledge of life, even when coming into a caring profession at an early age.

All of us, in the early years, have lived as part of a family group living within and relating to a particular community. Later, through education and other choices, we have participated in a wider range of small community groups in which the personality, the 'spiritual person', is developed. That person is unique with his or her own set of experiences, beliefs and understandings, all of which contribute to shaping the person and to the resource brought to the caring situation.

There has already been a very major input of learning and personal experience for each of us. Although there are different schools of thought about the nature of these early influences in the formative years of life, psychologists and sociologists alike are convinced of their importance in shaping our personalities.

Environmental influences appear to have the greatest effect during the periods of most rapid growth. It is thought that as much development occurs in the first 4 years of life as in the following 13 years. About 50% of intellectual growth takes place between birth and the fourth year of life, while 30% occurs between 4 and 8 years, (Kellner Pringle, 1975). It seems that children respond more readily to some experiences during certain critically sensitive phases of development.

The reader may find the different schools of thought somewhat conflicting but they can bring understanding to the whole concept of personality formation. The psychoanalytical approach has often concentrated on the importance of early bonding processes and attachment in infancy. While these may be controversial issues, it is generally recognised that they do play a part in establishing the capacity to form relationships in later life (Rutter, 1972; Foss, 1975; Storr, 1981). Learning theorists concentrate more on the significance of stimulus and response and the development of behaviour patterns (Elkin, 1960; Rogers, 1967)

Sociologists tend to take yet another perspective on socialisation processes as they consider the influences of families (primary socialisation), and of groups and cultural influences (secondary socialisation) on the formation of personality (White, 1977). Other key concepts for them are status and role theory, as well as class and cultural differences. There are interesting traditional associations apparent between religion and social class, which, in turn, influence lifestyle and behaviour patterns (Brothers, 1971).

One interesting study carried out by Bernstein in the Sixties demonstrates the effects of social class and culture on the child's development of language and conceptual thought (Lawton, 1970). This can have implications on our ability to understand and communicate with others from backgrounds which differ from our own.

While these different approaches may seem confusing at first, they all complement each other and play a valuable role in helping us to gain a wider perspective on potential differences and their origins. They can help us towards recognition and acceptance of these individual differences, which are clearly established by a combination of hereditary and environmental factors, social and cultural influences in early life, and the quality of formation of secure relationships.

EXERCISE 9
Look back at the outline of your spiritual journey in Exercise 6 and draw a map of it. This helps to identify some of the major influences which have shaped your thinking. This can be a personal exercise leading up to Exercise 10 opposite.

SELF-ACCEPTANCE

To be a carer who is effective as a resource, we need to accept ourselves with the experiences through which we have lived already and to reflect upon them and understand as far as possible their influences upon us. We need to note the kind of family of which we have been a part, the gifts we have received from our family and the implications of possessing those gifts. Some of us will have lived with material plenty and others with very little. Some have grown up in an environment rich in philosophical thought and have been exposed to books, literature and higher education, while others will have had very little of that kind of encouragement. Each of us will have been exposed to particular aspects of cultural life and will have had exposure, to some degree, to other cultures in our own society and to snippets of societies from other countries through the media and books. We have also been exposed to attitudes of prejudice and disregard for the beliefs, faiths and cultures of others.

One factor of immense importance for the carer as a personal internal resource, as well as having access to external resource material and expertise, is how far they have experienced security and acceptance, being valued without prejudice and had their own thoughts and beliefs (no matter how mature or immature) respected and allowed. An interesting Swedish study has recently assessed a security model and demonstrated that the carers who were most able to communicate with patients about approaching death were shown to be individuals secure in themselves (Hedley and Sjoqvist, 1988). Carers with secure personalities were also able to contribute more effectively to staff and family relationships. A good working atmosphere, knowledge, and psychological and administrative support also contribute to a sense of security for staff.

THE CARER'S RESOURCES – KNOW YOURSELF

There is a further aspect of past experience that has particularly relevant implications for the way in which carers respond to spiritual need. At this point readers may find it helpful to explore some related issues for themselves. It might be useful to consider the questions below as a group exercise for discussion, or on your own, before reading further or when you reach the end of the Chapter.

The influences of cultural background and childhood experiences on personality have already been noted and religious experience in the early years of family life is a significant aspect of this. For example, there is a proven relationship between social class and denominational allegiance in the UK (Brothers, 1971). While there may be converts from those of British birth to religions other than Christian, most of the adherents to other major religions of the world in the UK are found among families of immigrant origin. It has also been observed that people of other faiths who join Christian churches often retain some of the ethnic religious customs they grew up with in their primary culture.

It is apparent that we all retain some effects from our early experiences which influence our attitudes, beliefs, values and practices. This may also have subtle effects on our prejudices, anxieties and uncertainties when responding to the needs of others. It is therefore important for carers to be aware of the possible influences that have shaped their own personal beliefs and attitudes. It is a useful exercise to identify these and to clarify personal beliefs on some of the major dilemmas common to all of us, and to set out those beliefs and also to acknowledge the areas where there is doubt and confusion. This is an extremely valuable exercise as it gives confidence to the carer to have a starting place and helps bring an awareness of possible areas which might create a threatening situation. Surprisingly, it often identifies new strengths and resources that were previously unrecognised.

EXERCISE 10 (FOR PERSONAL OR GROUP CONSIDERATION)
- What is the meaning of life? Is there any purpose in life?
- Why do people suffer? Is there any value in suffering?
- Why is life so unfair to people?
- What are some of your own strengths which you consider to be attributes in your profession? Write down a list of your personal skills.

It is a useful exercise to identify our own individual gifts, attributes and resources and to write them down. When a group of professional carers is asked do this exercise, a common response is one of stunned silence and blank looks. After a while, a few may venture diffident suggestions but it takes some encouragement for individuals to be able to accept that everyone has something of value to offer – indeed all will have the experience of their particular professional training with its specific skills. Eventually most will find something special they can offer any relationship – some particularly valuable resource to be cultivated and enhanced, which is a potential asset when seeking to develop relationships in the spiritual dimension. Some of the most important gifts and skills are those which are taken for granted and therefore may not be recognised. These include listening, loving, caring and the desire to help others.

Carers respond to need as the individuals they are and from the place where they have reached in themselves. Each one is a unique person with a different set of personal values and attributes, and a particular spiritual personality of their own thus bringing a very special and unique dimension to spiritual care. It is vital for the carer to be aware of their own beliefs and strengths as well as possible areas of vulnerability, as this is the resource they bring to each situation and where they start from in any relationship.

THE CARING RELATIONSHIP – A MEETING OF EQUALS

An important question which has to be faced by the carer in relating to the patient at depth and in this particular way is, 'How far am I able to allow others to hold views which not only differ from my own but which may perhaps be, in some respects, totally opposed to mine? Can I allow that and value that person's right to be themselves as I hope to be accepted as myself?'

It is essential for the carer that when he or she comes alongside as a resource, it is to be a meeting of equals. It is perhaps of even greater importance that the relationship is one in which the carer is prepared to give up the control of the interaction into the hands of the person being cared for. The carer must be prepared to accept that person's agenda, and realise that their journey at that moment is more important than their own.

This is a concept of fundamental importance to the reader approaching spiritual care and one that is perhaps difficult for some carers to appreciate. A study of the excellent and comprehensive range of publications recently produced in relation to a range of aspects concerning spiritual care show this approach is conspicuous by its absence. There is little reference to addressing the patient's or client's 'felt' needs or to a 'partnership relationship' or consumer participation in defining what spiritual care is needed. Concentration remains on delivery of care with the carer giving the definitions and the parameters of normative need (Bradshaw, 1972). Some writers give anecdotal accounts of their own observations on how the patient or client feels (Bowers, 1990; Veness, 1990), but it was a rare discovery to find a counsellor writing a paper starting from an account of his own personal experience and spiritual journey, (Rowan, 1990).

This is not really so surprising when we consider the recent emphasis on 'delivery of care' in other fields, and similar observations were noted by the team studying the Marie Curie Nursing Service (Owen *et al.*, 1989, p. 48). Most of the criteria for defining need were set out by the carers, and there was little reference in the studies researched to patient participation in the caring team or to what the patient really felt about what he needed or would like.

Although we cannot entirely step aside from our own journey, there is great merit in the gift of being able to step aside momentarily and change direction and to walk along with the other person. One of the gifts much needed here is to be able to see the situation through the other person's eyes and to recognise the pain, without leaping to simplistic answers or responses, with a willingness to be exposed to that pain and to enter into it in a way which incorporates our own suffering with a willingness to embrace their suffering. So it is important for us to establish from the beginning that we are looking at a meeting of equals in a caring relationship and to remember that this approach is fundamental to all our consideration of spiritual care. The patient or client is thus also a resource for the carer, as without him there could be no dialogue and no meaningful caring relationship.

Staying

Through a caring committed presence people will discover:
That they are allowed to be themselves:
That they are loved and so are lovable.
That they have gifts, and their lives have meaning
That they can grow and do beautiful things
and in turn be peacemakers in a world of conflict.

Jean Vanier – *Journey to Wholeness*

QUESTION 1

a) How do you describe a 'relationship of equals'? Illustrate your answers by examples from your own experience.
b) What are the difficulties for professionals in establishing this relationship?

Key points

- The carer is a valuable resource in any caring relationship.
- Kindness and caring may be confused, although kindness is part of caring.
- Each carer brings a unique set of resources to the relationship.
- Environmental and cultural influences have a significant effect on shaping personality, attitudes and prejudices.
- A study of the evidence available can help us to understand ourselves.
- Self-acceptance and knowing oneself are important for the carer to become an effective resource.
- The carer's response is influenced by the kind of person he or she is.
- The caring relationship is a meeting of equals – a partnership.
- The carer may need to 'step aside' from his own journey to meet the other person where he is and walk along with him, sharing the situation just where the patient is.
- A fundamental aspect of spiritual care is that it is built on establishing a relationship of equals.

The carer's response to spiritual need – a relationship of equals

THE BASIS OF DIALOGUE

If you wish to enter the world of those who are broken
or closed in on themselves – it is important to
learn their language.

Jean Vanier – *The Broken Body*

ESTABLISHING A RELATIONSHIP

For the carer to respond to spiritual need, it is clear that the first step is to establish a relationship of trust with the patient and then to identify the needs. So often in the field of spiritual or religious care, the starting point appears to be that the carer has the answers ready packaged and is coming to deliver what he or she thinks the patient needs to assist him or her in the process of recovery. This clearly devalues the individuality of the patient or client, and places the carer's agenda above that of the person cared for, thus creating a hierarchical relationship.

We would certainly feel unhappy when visiting our GP as a patient if we saw the doctor writing out our prescription as we entered the door of the surgery. It is obvious that some kind of consultancy process should take place and a most important first step is to establish a relationship of trust between the doctor and the patient. We would then want the doctor to listen to us to hear about our symptoms. This may involve some questioning to eliminate certain factors and to discover the nature of the situation. A careful examination may then be necessary and the findings together with the doctor's experience, knowledge, and understanding assist in arriving at a diagnosis. This is followed by a response in the form of explanation and prescription of the appropriate treatment. Surely the same level of perception and respectful care is required when delivering spiritual care.

Another important aspect of this is to make the patient feel comfortable in the presence of the carer. For those responsible for the delivery of care, an important stepping stone may be to relieve immediate suffering of a physical nature. Those who deliver hands-on care often have an unrecognised advantage by having the first level of trust established through a good professional response to pain and physical distress.

For those offering hands-on care, this aspect needs to be fully developed and those without this advantage need to find other ways of establishing rapport with their patient that can be perceived by the patient as valuing him or her as a person and not simply as a condition or disease.

THE FIRST MOVES – GETTING COMFORTABLE

The first step is to find out and use, with respect, the name by which the patient prefers to be addressed. The number of patients called by a name which no one ever uses for them outside of the hospital is amazing. Many patients feel unable to challenge the automatic use of their first name as it appears on the admission form or indeed to ask to be called 'Mr' or 'Mrs' if that is the form of address preferred. It should be remembered that to be called by an unfamiliar name that irritates may well cause further distress and discomfort to a person who is already feeling uncomfortable and threatened by their situation which could cause feelings of alienation.

> *Call me by my own familiar name, speak*
> *to me in the easy way ... wear no false*
> *air of solemnity or sorrow ... Let my name be*
> *ever the household word it ever was.*

Henry Scott Holland 1847–1918, Canon of St Paul's Cathedral

Developing communication skills that enable the carer to help the patient to feel comfortable and at ease is a gift to that patient and may help reverse feelings of being in an uncomfortable and alien environment. We must never forget that, from the earliest moments of our lives, we have naturally and automatically turned to human beings for assurance and comfort when in distress. (The skills needed for this kind of care will be dealt with in more detail in Chapters 5 and 6.)

The establishment of a comfortable relationship and rapport makes it possible for further sharing of the situation to take place. In order to know how to respond to need it must be recognised, acknowledged and shared. The carer needs to recognise that the patient had a life before becoming a patient and entering hospital and hopefully will continue to have a life after his stay is over. He has both family and friends, working skills, a social status and life, interests and hobbies. By coming into hospital anxieties, fears, doubts and concerns develop, which amount to depersonalisation of the individual.

Example

The following incident in a casualty department illustrates this point. One very cold night in winter when it was snowing heavily outside, a patient who had been admitted kept on saying 'Snow, snow – my poor snow, snow". The staff kept saying 'Yes, yes – you are in the warm now, you'll be alright'. It took them a while to realise he was talking about his dog named 'Snowy' who was left tied to a railing near the place where the patient had collapsed.

Being able to help a person feel comfortable is a very powerful tool. Just as it is difficult to share anything in depth with someone in extreme pain where the first need is to relieve that pain, so too a person feeling alienated and uncomfortable needs to be made mentally and spiritually at ease in order to have the confidence and the ability to share deeper thoughts and questions of hope, fear and doubt.

THE CARER'S RESPONSE – COMING ALONGSIDE

Carers who are prepared to enter into this kind of helping relationship, as we have seen in the last Chapter, need to be aware of their own vulnerability and strengths in terms of meeting pain and suffering. The response of the carer is not primarily in words but in coming alongside patients, listening, hearing what they want to say, and above all staying with them. This means a level of commitment that cannot just be abandoned when the going gets tough and may need the involvement of a team to provide continuity of care in depth (*see Chapter 16*). With someone to share the darkest experience, the patient may well find the despair and hopelessness begins to clear with the realisation that they have been heard in the deepest place where they feel most threatened, the outlook begins to change. This is something similar to passing through a very long tunnel. There is a point near the centre where the darkness is at its most intense and feelings of disorientation are strongest. Moving into the tunnel is an experience of deepening and oppressive darkness engulfing the person. Then a small circle of light appears ahead and gradually grows bigger until the darkness recedes behind. The ever growing circle of light always lies ahead.

Patients in the depth of despair and hopelessness may experience that first glimmer of light when someone has come alongside them in a way that enables them to feel heard in the deepest and darkest place of their being. Having someone to share the experience makes it feel safer and less threatening. Often words are not the appropriate response – it is never helpful for the carer to respond even by saying 'I understand', but simply receiving the shared experience may bring a reassurance that words fail to bring. So the first response of the carer, once comfort has been ensured, is to be prepared to listen and to receive whatever the patient wishes to share.

EXERCISE 11

Every professional will have a range of possibilities to draw on when endeavouring to put another person at ease. It is a valuable exercise to explore ways in which each different professional carer in your group would do this.

Learning a language
is learning what people are really saying.
The non-verbal as well as the verbal language....
You must go deeper....
And discover what it means
to listen deeply to another....
in order to understand people both in their pain and in their grief, to
understand what they are really asking so that you can hold their wound,
their pain and all that flows from it....
You must go deeper and discover what it really means to see another–
To see the light shining in the darkness –
To give another hope and trust.

Jean Vanier – *The Broken Body*

SOME CHALLENGES FOR THE CARER

Such relationships, however, can create a very exposed situation for the carer, which can prove threatening. At this point there is often a temptation to step aside and to deal with more tangible and practical issues. These seem easier to the carer as they are more satisfying and bring a sense of achievement of accomplishment. This may bring frustration to a patient, however, when he realises he has not been heard. The problem-solving approach may be a way of stopping the process when the situation becomes too threatening. This may feel safer and more comfortable to the carer but is less helpful to the patient.

Professional carers may often have a strong desire to comfort the patient by saying, 'Don't be frightened, there is always hope'. It is tempting to offer reassurance and there may be a strong urge to do this in religious terms, which is an apparently easier approach and perhaps more conventional, as well as serving to reinforce the carer's own security. In fact, the patient may well know there is no real substance or truth in the reassurance and will soon realise the carer is simply unable to face the intensity of fear, distress and reality that exists. The patient will avoid sharing painful feelings in future. This is why it is essential for carers to be aware of their own personal areas of vulnerability, and to be able to acknowledge that they are permissible. It helps to realise that all that is required is to listen without trying to explain or to reassure. It may be helpful for the patient to accept that professional carers do not have ready answers to cope with suffering and death as the patient may know deep down that there are no answers, but still have a deep need to ask and explore the questions.

This is where the carers need to have ready access to support for themselves and this will be looked at in more depth later in this book. Such an experience of vulnerability in offering spiritual care may prove to be a period of personal growth and development for the carer. If adequate support and encouragement is available at the time, it enables them to return to the situation using new insights and ready to explore the new territories with greater confidence.

COPING WITH PERSONAL ANXIETIES FOR THE CARER

That there are often no clear answers to give is a common difficulty for many professionals in offering spiritual care. It may lead to negative responses in the form of dismissing the problem or distancing themselves from the patient through practical activity as described above. The exploratory approach may be particularly difficult for someone with a very explicit faith of their own who may experience a sense of personal guilt or failure when answers cannot be given and accepted.

The difficulty grows where the patient is unable to come through to a sense of peace or acceptance of the situation. A great deal of maturity is needed for the carer to realise that the fear and anger of the patient is an indication that the skills offered in providing spiritual care have enabled him or her to acknowledge the reality of his or her emotions. It may be that healing and a sense of peace will follow in the knowledge that these emotions have been accepted. Some patients, however, may never come to a place of peace or acceptance and they remain fearful, angry and anxious to the end. This does not necessarily mean the carer has failed.

Some carers also have difficulty in respecting the patient's rights to receive the kind of spiritual care appropriate to their beliefs in whatever manner they are accustomed to, when this differs from the carer's own beliefs and principles. There may be a need to bring in a representative of the patient's own faith to give a form of care alien to the carer. It is not always easy to acknowledge that others may see facets of the truth which differ from our own perceptions and to give a proper respect to their views. It may help carers to have a less infallible view of truth if we look back and recognise that our view of truth has changed in the light of growing experience.

> *Our highest truths are but half truths.*
> *Think not to settle down for ever in any truth.*
> *Make use of it as a tent in which to pass a summer night*
> *But build no house of it or it will be your tomb.*
>
> J J Balfour – Quoted from Bishop Mervyn Stockwood

Another response that needs to be modified in some situations arises from the assumption that complete cure or freedom from symptoms is the only satisfactory outcome following good care. We know this is not possible in some cases and our response will need to be adjusted in line with the reality of the situation if we are to be able to come alongside and stay with the patient in offering spiritual care. This adaptation is not easy in a world where professional carers are conditioned to consider that complete cure is the ultimate satisfactory conclusion.

EXERCISE 12
This is probably best as a personal exercise. Identify some fears, doubts and personal feelings you have experienced yourself in dealing with patients' anxieties about their own situations. Later you may wish to look at these in a group setting and share in some of the ways in which other professionals have approached these situations.

THE CARING RELATIONSHIP – A PARTNERSHIP

Throughout the discussion in this Chapter we have assumed that the concept of a 'partnership' is a key aspect in this caring relationship. It is apparent, however, that this idea has a wide range of interpretations amongst carers and the literature on this subject is very limited (Bayntum-Lees, 1992). A comprehensive review of studies on home care for terminally ill patients found many references to team care and lip service given to the patient's needs but only one study actually referred to the patient being involved in team decisions relating to his or her own care (Owen *et al.*, 1989).

Baynton-Lees (1992), in her study on nurses, points out that, while nurses believe intuitively that a partnership relationship is ideal, there are difficulties in incorporating this concept into their own belief systems. She stresses the need not only for understanding, but also for a fundamental change in attitudes and thinking patterns towards care. Other writers refer to the importance of self-awareness in the carer in such a therapeutic encounter.

There is a delicate balance between power or control, on the one hand, and mutual commitment and equality, on the other, within a reciprocal relationship. This is best achieved in a comfortable atmosphere of trust and acceptance as discussed earlier in this Chapter. It is important to remember, however, that although this concept gives patients the right to make their own choices or the power to join in making decisions, some may prefer not to be involved in such responsibilities. Great sensitivity is required on the part of the carer and this often means just 'being with' the patient rather than 'doing things to them' (Muetzel, 1988). Muetzel's model of activities and factors in the partnership of caring is helpful to consider here.

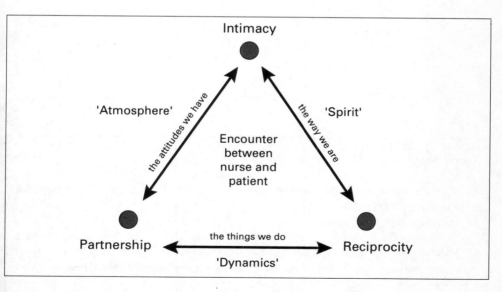

Muetzel's model of activities and factors in the partnership of caring (Muetzel 1988).

THE SKILLS INVOLVED WITH RESPONSE

The carers response to spiritual need requires a considerable level of professional skill and personal maturity and may therefore present a very threatening situation to many who would genuinely like to be involved. It is encouraging to know that there are some areas where carers may have natural insights or skills in offering this kind of care and just need encouragement and reinforcement to extend and develop these attributes. Alternatively, skills can be learned through teaching and practical experience, and more attention will be given to this later on in this section. The skills of communication, listening and using questions appropriately are practical examples of skills that can be acquired. Knowing how and when to use them wisely may encourage the process of exploration for the patient. Good observational skills are an asset that most professionals have acquired and are valuable when seeking for sensitivity to an individual's spiritual needs.

In summing up the carer's response, it is good to be reminded of Cicely Saunders' words: 'watch with me "means above all, just" "be there" ', (Saunders, 1965). Dugan says ,' '...the human spirit does not need judgments, advice or exhortations to change. It needs acceptance, listening, and the opportunity to be heard and understood: compassionate human contact. The human spirit needs to communicate in symbolic language', and he gives a useful method of structuring an 'atmosphere of open communication' (Dugan, 1987).

Key points

- The carer's response is determined by the parameters of the relationship established with the patient.
- This relationship is based on mutual trust and equality.
- The process is facilitated by simple measures such as establishing a comfortable environment, and coming alongside the person – just being there.
- Such a relationship may raise challenges for the carer that are threatening and give rise to personal anxieties.
- A partnership needs self-awareness, understanding, sensitivity and mutual respect.
- This requires the development of communication and listening skills.

CHAPTER 5

The carer's skills – looking, listening and communicating

The basis of dialogue
If you wish to enter the world of those who are broken and closed in on themselves – it is
important to learn their language...
You must go deeper and discover what it really means to see another
– to see the light shining in the darkness
– to recognise the seeds of hidden gifts . . .
– to give one another hope and trust, acceptance of his or her essential beauty
and to welcome their riches as they unfold

Jean Vanier – *The Broken Body*

The last Chapter touched on some of the ways in which the carer's response can be enhanced by special skills and in this Chapter some of the more practical aspects of those skills will be considered, together with the acquisition of skills. The following Chapter looks at the use of skills in assessment of spiritual need. When establishing rapport with a patient and entering into a relationship of trust as described earlier, a range of different communication skills can be used in the approach to spiritual care.

COMMUNICATION SKILLS

Communication skills involve a great deal more than simply talking to a person or passing on information. There are three major elements involved:
- The source of communication, which is the person giving information.
- The message to be transmitted or the communication to be shared.
- The recipient or person receiving the communication.

The process, however, is not as simple as just giving information; for it to be successful it must be received and understood as intended. This is a complex process, involving a range of variables and skills. For example, the person communicating and the recipient may have very different perceptions and expectations governed by their own experiences or may simply have language differences! Response, in turn, will be governed by the carer's ability to present the message in a way that can be understood and by the patient's capacity to receive, interpret and respond to information. One common example is when fear can have such a paralysing effect that any unpleasant news a person does not want to hear may be completely rejected and not registered at all (Kretch *et al.*, 1962).

Communication skills involve a thoughtful approach along the lines already discussed, helping the patient to feel comfortable and relaxed. Verbal skills are not the only ones to be used. Other skills that are helpful are listening, good eye contact, and observation of body language and facial expression or any manifestation of fear or tension. These skills involve using many of the senses.

The appropriate use of touch, and the awareness of the patient's response to this is a valuable skill. Counselling skills are valuable and some carers may have a particular insight and an aptitude for this which can be enhanced by further training. Another frequently overlooked skill is the capacity to remain silent, which is often the most helpful response when answers do not exist or when someone is working their own way through a difficult situation. It is important to remember that the approach used is an integrated one involving the use of a range of skills. No single skill is used in isolation to the exclusion of others.

VERBAL SKILLS

The obvious means of communication is through the use of language and it follows that it is essential for two people establishing a relationship to understand each other's language. The barrier of understanding a foreign language may not be the only one to face here: sometimes people who share the same nationality have difficulty with local accents or expressions and particularly with colloquial terms. This could be especially the case where religious practices and spiritual needs are concerned, so carers need to be alert and aware of this aspect. Professional staff also need to be particularly careful about the use of colloquialism or jargon, which may be a deterrent for some people who are afraid to ask for an explanation – alternatively, they may misinterpret the message. If the information given is important, it helps to create an opportunity for the recipient to repeat what they have understood from the carer.

If a real language barrier exists, the use of interpreters may not be helpful where spiritual care is concerned as the relationship is a vital element of the caring process and it may be advisable to call in a leader or other acceptable person of the patient's own nationality to assist the carer and share some of the responsibility.

> 'Write that down,' the king said to the jury and the jury
> eagerly wrote down all three dates on their slates and then
> added them up, and reduced the answer to shillings and pence.

Lewis Carroll – *Alice in Wonderland*

Asking questions

Many carers will be used to using a 'history taking' approach when seeking information from patients, without realising that this can have a depersonalising effect because it has a preconceived kind of photo-fit outcome which can be very misleading when trying to assess the kind of individual spiritual care needed. It is possible to make an assessment of spiritual need and of the care required without using this approach, by using open questions rather than leading or prescriptive ones.

A more oblique kind of questioning, if used, has better results. For example, rather than asking a direct question such as 'How many children do you have?', it would be more helpful to say, 'Are you expecting visitors today?' and this will open a conversation about family and friends. Most people will relax and talk easily about their families if approached in this way, leading on very naturally to more information about themselves, their values, beliefs and lifestyle. This approach is often known as the indirect question approach.

Open questions are another way of triggering a conversation, for example, 'How are you feeling about the treatment?' allows for a genuine response. In contrast, 'Was the treatment awful?' or 'You slept well last night didn't you?' are both leading or closed questions as they suggest what the answer should be and may get the answer they deserve! Leading questions can also have a tendency to 'programme' the answers required by making statements and adding something like, 'I'm sure you agree'.

There is a further type of question to be used with discretion. This is the probe question, which is probably best reserved for a well-established relationship at times when it is helpful to extend the person's thinking into new territory. For example, a question like, 'Have you been able to think about your situation yet?' could later be followed by, 'How can I help you in this?' enabling the patient to begin to work out an approach which he knows he can handle.

EXERCISE 13
- Jeremy is a 7-year-old patient in the burns unit with extensive burns on his limbs and trunk. He is restless, distressed and frightened by his situation and feeling very miserable.
- Louisa is an 83-year-old lady who has lived an active social life and is still intellectually lively. She recently had a stroke and lost the power of speech and is unable to write.
- Gita is a 25-year-old Pakistani girl who has been admitted for minor surgery. She is both deaf and dumb.

Consider these three patients and discuss among yourselves how you would:
  (a) Identify their spiritual need.
  (b) Communicate with them in the process of providing spiritual care.
  (c) Involve their families in their spiritual care.

Answering questions

Spiritual care is an area which poses the kind of questions where there are few straightforward answers. Sometimes the person asking questions knows there are no answers but needs the pain, fear and doubt of his questioning to be heard and accepted. Here, just listening and accepting what is expressed is the best approach. The kind of questions that revolve around the deeper meaning of life often appear with the onset of illness bringing uncertainty and insecurity. They are questions like:

'Why should this happen to me? I've hurt no one.'; 'Why should I be ill? I've done nothing wrong.'; 'Am I going to get well? Can I cope with illness?'; 'I've not had a chance to do anything worthwhile with my life yet, why should I be ill? I'm too young.' Other questions revolve around the family: 'Who is looking after the family? How will they manage? Will they know what is happening?'

Sometimes the questioner moves on to face life and death questions directly where there are no easy answers: 'What is life all about?' 'Is there any meaning to life?' 'If there is a God, why does he allow suffering?'

> *I said to the Heart 'How goes it?' Heart replied 'Right as a Ribstone Pippins.' But it lied.*
>
> Hilaire Belloc – *Epigrams*

Listening and hearing

Listening and hearing the pain which lies behind the questions is the baseline from which to start and just to 'be there' helps.

> *Those who listen day after day....in exposing themselves to another's pain are part of the healing process.*
>
> Sheila Cassidy – *Good Friday People*

Example

Sometimes just to pose a further question may help. One student nurse heard her patient ask the young registrar a direct question, 'Doctor, I'm dying am I not?' The doctor went very pink and quietly turned round and walked out unable to face this situation. The nurse was left unable to retreat. She stood quietly for a moment then asked, 'Why do you ask – are you afraid of dying?'. Her answer, 'Yes' came directly. Quickly the nurse responded, 'That makes two of us then', and the elderly patient sat up abruptly and said, 'Oh nurse, we can't have you afraid – you are far too young and precious', and they both laughed quietly and the conversation was opened up. Discussing this later with a tutor, the student explained that she had to go away afterwards and work out her own views on life and death but she then felt much more confident about facing these questions and moving along, starting with the patient.

There is more to 'hearing the real need' and this is explored more fully under the discussion on assessment skills.

EXERCISE 14
Consider how you would have answered this question, whether you were the medical registrar, nurse or physiotherapist.

THE CARER'S COPING SKILLS

Dealing with questions of such importance to the individual may well present a considerable challenge to many carers. It will draw heavily on their personal skills of coping and on their perception of what is really being communicated. These questions may well present a threat as they deal with life-and-death issues, which carers may never have had to face or consider for themselves. The patient's uncertainties may present themselves accompanied by a range of emotions such as anger, rejection, tears or refusal to cooperate. This, in turn, can generate reciprocal feelings of anxiety, anger and uncertainty in the carer and result in defensive behaviour such as avoiding the patient, rejection, defence and withdrawal from the situation.

For this reason, it is vital that all professional carers are given adequate preparation for coping with spiritual need and that proper support is available for all staff during the course of care. This kind of preparation and support will be dealt with later. It is an essential prerequisite for the development of skills needed for coping in these situations.

INTERPRETIVE SKILLS

Interpretive skills are necessary to bring together the range of observations made through other channels. A difficult area arises when good supportive skills have been used effectively to establish a good rapport and partnership which have worked well. The individual is then free to release some of the feelings which have hitherto been carefully controlled and repressed. When released, such feelings can pour out in a very powerful way as anger, fear, despair, rejection or withdrawal. This can leave the carer feeling very vulnerable and, at times, totally inadequate or a failure.

Here we are caught up in our own limitations or inhibitions, and in those learned responses, which we are often aware we have acquired from our past. For example, we may cope with anger by rejection because we have been rejected in the past for inappropriate behaviour when expressing anger. This kind of rejection may have led us to believe that such expression of anger is wrong and unacceptable in our culture. The expression of pain or tears of emotion can often cause painful embarrassment for both parties in a relationship. It also brings an additional threat in that the person and the situation appear to be out of control. This does not easily fit into the caring professional's image and the projected role of containing pain and emotion which is called controlling or managing the situation.

If the carer is disabled by such an expression and attempts to backtrack or to take control of the situation, the patient may be in a worse state; having viewed the chaos underneath revealing the pain, hopelessness and despair and receiving a response that is unable to cope with it or rejects it as legitimate behaviour. Such responses are frequently caused by the carer's feelings of anxiety, or inadequacy.

To facilitate a creative response to such an unloading and opening up of repressed feelings requires the carer to accept the attitudes and responses of the individual in the painful circumstances they are experiencing, whatever their nature. It needs the ability to be with, and to stay with, the person in order to enable them to explore the pain they so much dread and to verbalise the questions which may well lead to yet more questions. The carer needs to avoid the desire to bring in tidy answers.

The carer's role here is an enabling one and not a teaching role or one giving information (although this often feels more reassuring for the carer!). For the experience to be of any value, the patient needs to discover for himself the understanding which may indicate the way forward on this part of the journey and own them for himself as his own creation. As we saw earlier in this book, the carer is there to accompany the patient on his journey and to help in avoiding the pitfalls. Any move or attempt to fit or push them into a straitjacket response is not going to assist them through the experience.

> So when you are listening to somebody completely,
> attentively – then you are listening not only to the words
> but also to the feeling of what is being conveyed, to the
> whole of it, not part of it.

J Krishnamurti

Key points

- Particular skills are involved in the carer's approach to spiritual care.
- Good communication skills are essential and need an understanding of the complex processes involved.
- An understanding of the complexity of the processes of suffering is needed.
- Communication skills include verbal and tactile skills, listening skills and the skill to observe and to interpret.
- Interpretive skills need sensitivity and awareness.
- The carer's role is an enabling one.

CHAPTER 6

The carer's assessment skills –
putting it all together

Write that down' the king said to the jury, and the
jury eagerly wrote down all three dates on their slates, and
then added them up, and reduced the answer to shillings and pence.

Lewis Carroll – *Alice in Wonderland*

Before attempting to respond to spiritual need, it must first be recognised and assessed. It is essential to see the person not just as a patient and to listen to each person, identifying and hearing their real need. It is all too easy to be sidetracked and to concentrate on what is happening to the patient, rather than seeing or hearing the person themselves. It is also easy to make an assessment by a preconceived measure or standard assessment of suffering based on the condition, illness or treatment being given to the patient or client. There may be a much greater need, deeper pain or suffering for a person having a relatively minor operation or procedure than for a person in the adjoining bed going through a major operation or treatment.

Suffering strikes at the core of the being and can be deeply penetrating or of incredible intensity when there is no physical pain present. At times we may be misled into thinking that we have dealt with suffering when in reality we have only dealt with the physical pain.

Assessment skills are essential in identifying spiritual need and thus enabling the most appropriate provision of spiritual care. Discussion of these skills must be seen within the context of a range of communication skills involving the use of all our senses together with a high level of sensitivity. Each individual carer contributes their own uniqueness as a person and also contributes their own set of skills to this situation. Some of these are intuitive and some acquired by experience and practice.

A FRAMEWORK FOR SPIRITUAL SKILLS

Assessment of spiritual need is probably one of the most ignored aspects of assessment and only in very recent years have any formal models been suggested in this field. On the whole, these tend to be more specifically concerned with religious need. One or two writers suggest that, for nurses, this is dealt with within the context of the nursing process.

Example

The model most often quoted is a guide put forward by Stoll in 1979. He offered four areas for spiritual appraisal to identify various aspects of spiritual concern including:

- The person's concept of God or deity.
- The person's source of strength and hope.
- The significance of religious practices and rituals.
- The perceived relationship between the client's spiritual beliefs and his or her state of health (Stoll, 1979).

Clifford (1987) suggests these areas provide a framework for formulating a spiritual assessment tool, but gives no further enlightenment on how this tool might be developed. A more detailed set of criteria for using Stoll's model can be found in a paper by Burkhardt *et al.* (1985), which includes suggestions for observing the individual's response to his situation in terms of responses like fear, guilt and hopelessness. Their discussion is quite useful, but again the emphasis is mostly on religious criteria.

Models can be useful tools for helping to identify areas of need as long as they are seen as a framework which can be modified or expanded. They should not be used in a prescriptive way, which has a danger of moulding the patient's progress to the model rather than the model being used to enhance the understanding of the personal experience.

USING OUR EYES

Our eyes are one of the most important assessment tools we have at our disposal. They are also one of the ways in which we communicate care and understanding. Looking at a patient, and indeed the way we look at them as we approach the bed, is of the utmost importance no matter what we have come for. It is so easy to be trapped in a professional tunnel vision as our eyes move immediately to the drip, the monitor, or to the part of the person's body to be dealt with.

Treatment can be transformed so easily by beginning with the person; meeting the eyes in good eye-to-eye contact accompanied by facial expression showing that we are seeing a person who is of value, and not just another patient in a numbered bed. Such contact begins to set the scene for a genuine meeting in which real need can be expressed freely. Eyes are a powerful means of communication, which is a reason why film-makers often use close-ups of eyes on screen at critical or poignant moments when words alone are inadequate.

The importance of this contact, which is often referred to as 'the meeting of the eyes', is confirmed by its wide recognition in literature and classical art forms down the centuries. Taylor (1972) calls it: 'the seeing which is not observation but encounter.' He continues: 'The fact that .... someone is there suddenly becomes important ...it commands attention ... the mutual recognition of seer and seen'.

In such moments of encounter we become aware of the real truth of each other. This kind of encounter is a basic skill for any real assessment of spiritual need.

Even in a fleeting moment, important messages may be transmitted, which can then lead on, at an appropriate time, to sharing at depth. For example, catching a glimpse of fear or loneliness, hopelessness or despair – perhaps noticing the tears quickly brushed aside, the look of longing, the mixture of hope and desperation, mute questioning such as: 'Can you really see me, really understand what is happening to me ? Do you care ? Will you stay with me? Can I trust you? Can I lean on you or rely on you? Can you see how desperate I am?'

All of this and much more can be expressed in a fleeting second of eye contact and if we do not look into those eyes we shall never see the unspoken cries for help. On the other hand, eyes can be equally offputting. To stare at or, to avert the eyes can create great tension. To look coldly and appraisingly without underlying care simply closes doors or creates uncertainty such as, 'They don't care about me' or 'What are they hiding from me?', Even worse, it can put in place defence mechanisms which may fool the professional into thinking 'This person has no special needs...'.

Once having arrived at the bedside it is important to position ourselves in such a way that eye contact can be engaged in a manner that lets the patient feel in control of such contact. Ideally, one needs to be at the side and looking in the same direction as the patient, which signifies 'being with' and also allows the patient to develop eye contact. There is a difference when carrying out a procedure or dressing, however, where we must be at the side or foot of the bed but where, because of engagement in that activity, momentary eye contact need not be threatening or overpowering.

At different times in the encounter the eyes transmit different messages and may be reinforced by changes in body posture, which might also indicate the patient's depth of need. Eye contact is normally the first person-to-person touch from carer to patient and, when allied to the use of touch and skill, may bring about a very close communication or rapport. Again if we are holding hands, various messages can be conveyed through the way in which the patient's hand is held and through changes

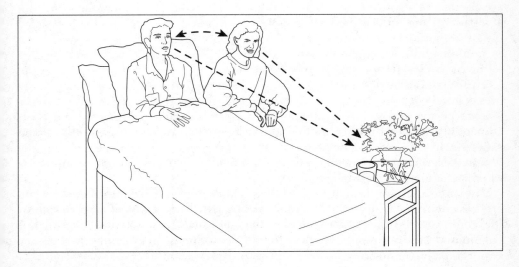

Listening to a patient.

in pressure used, which reinforces and emphasises the meaning given and received through words or tears. Touch may progress to holding where a very deep expression of pain, suffering, fear and need are expressed. Within that hold, a safety and security may be communicated, which enables the exploration of those needs.

EXERCISE 15

When you have read this section on eye contact, follow it up with some observations of your own. Notice how people in various situations such as your teachers and other professionals make eye contact, and write down some of your observations.

THE USE OF OTHER SENSES – PERCEPTION, TOUCH AND HEARING

The hands and body are important interpretive tools in helping us to hear and understand suffering and recognise need. Likewise our ears are important tools of assessment, especially when allied to a mind that is tuned in not just to listen to the words but to hear both what is on the surface and underneath. A mind so tuned will hear clues and cues given which indicate deeper needs and may fly completely in the face of surface protestations that everything is 'OK'. Being tuned in to such cues gives the carer the ability to hear when a person is portraying the role he or she believes is expected. Patients often perceive that they must adopt a role of appearing stoical, grateful and confident in the care offered. In addition, they feel they should appear to be coping well, for the sake of family and friends, while underneath the surface all is turmoil and fear.

PERCEIVING THE REAL PERSON

> *I said to Heart 'How goes it?'. Heart replied, 'Right as a*
> *Ribstone Pippins!' But it lied.*
>
> Hilaire Belloc – *Epigrams*

There are examples of this perceived role to be seen quite frequently when relatives tell professionals, often in the patient's hearing:

'He is a real fighter', or 'She will overcome all difficulties', or 'She is always an optimist – she won't let this defeat her.'

Recently a mother was heard to say of her teenage son, 'He's a brave lad – he won't cry,' just after he had been the victim of a stabbing incident – and he naturally felt he had to put on a brave appearance after that, although he was actually terrified. A person may have portrayed himself or herself to the family over the years as someone who is never down and never gives in. In such circumstances, there may be a need to create a time and a place for that person to be accepted in their anger and weakness with their tears and sadness. They may need permission to 'go off-duty' from that role for the time being.

The ears, helped by sensitivity and concentration, enable the throwaway word, phrase or sentence to be heard, registered and responded to at the appropriate moment. It is not only what is said in terms of actual words but also the tone of voice: the half-whispered question or exclamation; the tension, fear or resignation in the voice; over-confidence and over-emphasis. All of these can be heard by a good listener. This is all part of general listening skills and it involves the careful use of silence as mentioned below. The eyes, ears and sensitivity to responses need a mind that is ready and willing to hold the information received through these channels and to use it appropriately and at the right moment.

THE USE OF SILENCE IN ASSESSMENT

One of the rarely recognised skills of assessment is the ability to use silence – a silence which is comfortable, assuring and accepting, which allows safety for the person to continue an internal exploration of their needs. Often it is accompanied by touch and with the carer just staying there. This frequently allows the underlying situation to be looked at more fully in safety and to be appraised by the individual without him or her ever having to say very much openly. This iceberg situation is one where the patient may have showed the tip of the iceberg, but feels that they shared the whole of themselves with the other person and indeed may have communicated at depth.

> *A part of all art is to make silence speak*
> *The things left out in the painting*
> *The note withheld in music*
> *The void in architecture*
> *All are as necessary and as active as the utterance itself.*

Freya Stark – *The Zodiac Arch*

TOUCH AS PART OF ASSESSMENT

The skill of touch is a very important part of the carer's communication response and, as such, will be explored from several perspectives in this book. Firstly, it is widely accepted as a vital diagnostic tool and part of the diagnostic process in medicine to examine the patient, as in palpation, during pregnancy, abdominal examination or in assessing the range of movement of limbs after injury. Here it is usually used in conjunction with a stated history or recognised list of symptoms or other tests carried out and it plays a part in reaching a diagnosis.

Secondly, touch is a very powerful agent in the healing process when used by someone with healing skills or during the treatment given by a physiotherapist in massage to relieve pain. It can also be seen as a statement of contract when establishing a relationship, or used as an agent of control in manipulation, restraint or support when necessary.

So we are interested in touch as an assessment tool in looking at spiritual need and care and, as in the situations mentioned already, it plays an important part, together with other observations in arriving at a composite picture from which an accurate assessment may be made.

MESSAGES CONVEYED THROUGH TOUCH

Very strong messages can be communicated and strong pictures built up by touch. A good example is the use of touch by a blind person to establish in their own minds a picture and understanding of the person they are with.

Perhaps the most widely used and accepted form of touch in spiritual care will be the holding of a person's hand. The very way in which the hand is held can carry very important information. There is the fearful hold, gripping in this intensity, despairingly clinging on to a straw of security; the grip of pain from which release is sought by a firm grip; the grip of hopelessness, where there is no life in the hold and a statement of giving up is conveyed; the grip of determination to fight; and the peaceful hold which says 'I have come to terms with where I am, I welcome your presence and am pleased to know you are there but I don't need help right now' (Feltham, 1991; Dickleman, 1992).

Detailed pictures of the individual may be built up by combining the information communicated through eyes, ears, silence and touch. Deep levels of feeling can be experienced. At times the different aspects of communication will be complementary while at other times, they may become dissonant. There may be a move from a gentle hold to a more powerful grip as a fearful projection of a memory is relived. Sometimes a grip will convey a very different message from the words being spoken. Words might say 'I'm fine – I can cope, I don't need help' when the hand speaks of desperation and panic, and shouts 'Please help me!' Sometimes hands may say 'Please stay with me' when the words say 'You have to go now'.

Through touch and hold, a door is opened to the carer offering insights that otherwise might never be available. The message from the professional can now be understood as, 'I am recognising a person who is willing and waiting to hear you and to know who you are.'

EXERCISE 16
Mary is a blind patient and very frightened because she has just been told she had to face major surgery. Work through this exercise with a partner in your group, taking turns to be Mary and the carer. Record your impressions of the responses shared and the messages given and received as the news is given.

THE FRAMEWORK FOR ASSESSMENT

Thus it can be seen that a number of very basic tools can be used to build up a picture establishing who the person is and what some of their needs may be. If done well, these observations establish the patient's most basic personal needs requiring spiritual care. The purpose of the assessment will be to arrive at an overall picture and also to be able to identify where there are question marks and inconsistencies or clear statements of need.

A framework for assessment of spiritual need

The kind of observations that need recording will include:
* The person's concept or view of themselves.
* Their perception of what is happening to them.
* Their hopes, fears and natural support mechanisms.
* The strength and nature of support from family and friends.
* The nature of relationships within the family.
* Their own views and beliefs in relation to their situation.
* Their stated religion or commitment to religious practice.
* Their cultural background.
* Their life experience.
* An assessment of their natural defence and coping mechanisms.
* Their openness and receptivity to help.
* Assessment of their general state of health.
* Assessment of mental and emotional well being.

The way in which such observations are recorded may need to vary between individuals or indeed between different institutions. To lay out stereotyped questions for response may invite predetermined answers and so disguise or limit recognition of the real needs as presented. It should be possible, however, to give a clear picture of each individual using the above guidelines for recording assessments. (See also Burhardt *et al.*, 1994.)

In some cases the need for help may be well hidden and any support offered needs to be given with great sensitivity and in a subtle way without an obvious offer of help. In other situations, the need to regard the information received with total confidentiality may be uppermost. Nevertheless, it is important to be able to give support in such a way that the necessary care is provided. In other cases the demand is very open and the needs are more clearly stated.

QUESTION 1
Describe a situation you have dealt with which was particularly challenging and needed good communication skills. Explore ways in which you met the needs in this situation and ways in which other professionals might respond differently.

Key points

- Communication skills are basic tools for assessment of need.
- Various models have been suggested for use in this field.
- Models are useful tools but should be used with caution as a framework or guide to practice. Used with rigidity they can obscure real needs.
- Eye contact is an important skill. In the meeting of the eyes there is encounter, observation and the conveyance of messages.
- Observation leads to perceiving or seeing the 'real person'.
- Touch is a vital part of communication. It can be used for many purposes such as treatment, therapeutic care or to convey messages.
- Finally, a framework has been devised which can be used as a guide for making observations for assessment.

The carer's resources – sharing the load

No man can reveal to you aught but that which already lies
half asleep in the dawning of your knowledge.
The teacher who walks in the shadow of the temple, among
his followers, gives not of his wisdom but rather of his faith
and his lovingness.
If he is indeed wise he does not bid you enter the house of
his wisdom, but rather leads you to the threshold of your own mind.

Kahlil Gibran – *The Prophet*

Previous Chapters have explored various aspects of the carer's response to spiritual need, the factors influencing the nature of that response and the skills used in the process of responding to need and offering care. This chapter completes the circle by focusing on the range of resources available to the carer which he or she can rely upon to enhance personal skills and to facilitate the provision of spiritual care.

Exploration of the current literature available to assist carers in assessing their own resources in relation to the delivery of spiritual care reveals that little attention seems to be given to this aspect of preparation. Most writers are more concerned with identifying special areas of need or with looking at the nature of care and its delivery. That carers themselves are a constant and crucial element in the process seems to escape attention. Carers it seems are expected to find their resources elsewhere. Allen, for example, draws attention to this difficulty for nurses and points out that many are not comfortable with this aspect of care because they are so reticent about recognising this part of themselves and also what is missing is a language of spirituality with which they feel at home (Allen, 1991).

No individual carer is expected to come to the situation as a complete resource in themselves, or to act independently or alone in the process. Their skills and experience will be much more effective by knowing where support and complementary resources can be found and that the care can be shared. So this chapter attempts to draw together some of the important and relevant factors and to show that we are a resource in ourselves. In addition to the acquisition of skills as outlined in the previous chapters, there are other ways to complement these skills and resources and to equip ourselves to enhance our caregiving.

It will help to clarify our understanding of the resources available if they are looked at under four different headings:

(1) The resources within the individual and the process of developing those resources.

(2) The resources within the team in a specific professional discipline and also those in the wider interdisciplinary team working in the hands-on situation.

(3) The resources or expertise which can be brought in for a specific need in a particular situation.

(4) The wider support network available to enable the provision of spiritual care.

THE INDIVIDUAL'S RESOURCES

A very powerful element in the response to spiritual need must come from the individual who is there and chosen by the patient and family as someone in whom they have confidence and are prepared to trust to enter into their personal territory and share their deepest needs. Such a trust puts a considerable personal responsibility on carers as their response needs to be at a sufficiently high standard to be of genuine assistance. This is where confidence, together with the development of personal skills, is of the utmost importance.

The carer's personal gifts

The biggest resource of all and the one that can be given with great effect, so long as the carer has adequate support, is the gift of themselves: the gift of their attention, care, concern, sincerity and love. For a busy professional, to give time is seen as a gift by the patient. Frequently, patients hold back from seeking that gift because they feel staff are too busy or their needs are not sufficiently important to warrant time to be spent on them. So the ability to communicate care and understanding in a way that leads a person into a sharing relationship is vital. There needs to be an accompanying willingness and ability to stay exposed to personal pain and suffering. The gift of that time and attention, when given with care and concern, is healing in itself.

In Chapters 5–7, we explored some aspects of the carer's response and the skills of listening, touching and trying to hear what is being said. That all forms part of the basis for carers to see themselves as a resource to the patient simply by being there and drawing on those skills. This can be done by listening attentively, trying to hear what is beyond the words, tears or expressions and giving value by acceptance. The danger is to feel that the carer's only resource is to give specific treatment more related to the ability to accept and care. It is important, as we indicated earlier, for the carer to recognise and acknowledge the value of their own life experience. Understanding and belief, regardless of it being from a limited number of years in many cases, is valid. The gift of oneself is the most valuable resource any carer can offer.

The carer's beliefs

While personal beliefs should not be imposed upon others, the carer's beliefs have an influence over their attitudes and in some cases they may be asked to confirm those beliefs. When invited to share their beliefs, to do so without trying to impose it, is a legitimate course of action and can help the patient to see and meet with the real person in the carer. The carer who is open to learn recognises that the truth is something we are all seeking and struggling to understand, rather than a static commodity that cannot be changed. To seek together with the patient and to make new discoveries of truth is journeying together. To be dismissive of the views of others and to simply try to superimpose one's own is to attempt a 'take over'.

A second arm to the professional resource is the knowledge and understanding acquired through professional training which gives a basis of knowledge which expands and deepens with experience and further periods of study and reflection. While recognising the value of one's internal and personal resources, these need to be balanced by professional knowledge and skill.

EXERCISE 17
At this stage in the book you may find it useful to identify your personal gifts or skills and write them down. Next consider the resources and skills you would like to have available from other people. If you are working in a group, share these skills and resources and look at what you have within the group as a whole. This should help to identify the group's resources and strengths if working together as a team.

RESOURCES IN THE TEAM

At both the personal and professional level, it is always important to recognise our own limitations and to know when we have moved out of our depth. We can admit this openly and freely to the person concerned while continuing to offer care and understanding. At the same time, we can indicate other avenues and resources of care relevant to the identified need. Some assistance may well come from other members of the same profession. Consequently, we need to be aware of the value of different attributes and skills of other members of our own profession and we need to have the humility to know that no one person can be the right person for every patient and family all of the time. To link the patient and family with the right member of the team at the appropriate time is a vital skill for providing the highest quality of care for any professional.

At times it may not be obvious which member of the team is the right person to approach and we may find it wise to tap the combined wisdom of the group in identifying the most appropriate person or way of responding to the need. The wider implications are that there will be occasions when members of another profession will be required for some needs, and in some cases those who have had personal experience of a similar situation will be required. Examples of this can be found where there is special experience to be tapped in a stoma therapy group or in an ileostomy self-help group. Some professionals may have accumulated special experience through circumstances; for example, if they have been involved with debriefing following a major disaster, or if they have worked in another culture for a while and gained an insight into spiritual needs within that culture. (This is more fully developed in Section III and Chapter 16.)

THE CARER'S RESOURCES FOR SPECIFIC NEEDS

It is unfortunate that those who hold strong or extreme beliefs of their own sometimes find it hard to call in other resources. Those who hold very 'particularist' views find it especially hard to bring in someone who holds views which differ from their own. This is both an arrogant approach and poor care. One does not call in a physician because one believes in total everything that that physician believes. Other resources to draw in include psychologists, psychiatrists, social workers, chaplains or members of individual faith or culture groups. In the field of spiritual care, there needs to be as much care given to calling in an appropriate resource person to meet a particular need as when calling in any other therapist such as a speech therapist or occupational therapist.

In considering the delivery of spiritual care, it is not only those professionals in the medical/nursing team who are involved. As much weight should be given to the skills available and the contributions made from those in other professions such as physiotherapy, occupational therapy, speech therapy and a range of alternative therapies which are now increasingly recognised and valued.

Alternative therapies

As we are looking at spiritual care in terms of the care of the whole person, or holistic care, one important aspect is to give time and attention to the individual's particular needs and desires. There is a number of alternative treatments available today which have gained a wide publicity through the media and in some quarters have gained acceptance, while in other areas there is scepticism about their value. Any special preferences patients may have do need to be recognised if we are to offer the widest form of response to individual need. These alternatives range from therapies of longstanding practice which some people have found to be beneficial such as osteopathy, homeopathy or acupuncture, to the more recent popular additions including aromatherapy, reflexology, visual imagery, relaxation and meditation. Some of these are already frequently incorporated with current medical practice such as hypnosis (Rankin-Box, 1998; Stevenson, 1992).

There are several common facets involved with these therapies which have helped to establish them as valuable forms of treatment for some individuals. First, there is the basic principle of choice – the person has opted to seek that form of care and treatment given. This is a valuable principle in that it helps the person to re-establish responsibility for their own lives to some extent and to reinforce personal dignity and self-esteem.

Second, the majority of alternative therapies demand the establishment of a very personal relationship and the giving of one-to-one time, in a one-to-one situation. This may well convey a sense of being valued and lead to the recipient experiencing a deeper level of personal worth. An important element of the value offered by the therapist in almost all of these therapies is the association with touch in some form. The therapeutic value of touch and massage is widely recognised and has great value in making an important statement of acceptance, especially for a patient who feels in some way that they have become unacceptable to other people (McGlone, 1990; Oldfield, 1992).

Thus there is a certain 'feel-good factor' involved with all of these therapies which may not be measured in terms of cure but rather in enhanced quality of life. This principle is something which is being encouraged by the medical and nursing professions in particular these days as more attention is once again being given to activities that enhance quality of life, such as doing the patient's hair. Personal contact is a prominent feature in the delivery of some aspects of care as it has always been. Treatment such as a bedbath involves the personal attention of a professional for a length of time. Such personal aspects of care can easily be undervalued as technology develops and professional skills needed to handle new knowledge and equipment take precedence. This can be a cause of diversion from personal relationship aspects of care.

Very little research has been done to explore this 'feel-good factor'. If it is to be done, there is a need to investigate not only whether the therapy has produced a cure but to what extent the quality of life is enhanced. This obviously also applies to therapies like meditation and visualisation, which again involve the development of the individual's understanding and knowledge about themselves and their condition, but also encourage them to look outwards as well as inwards (Byrne, 1992).

In some of these therapies such as aromatherapy, there is a link into more than one of the senses. For example, if a patient has a condition associated with an unpleasant odour, aromatherapy can create a very pleasing response for a sense that has in some way been offended. This helps the individual to feel more acceptable, especially because someone has felt able to be with them, to touch them and enter into close personal contact.

Other aspects of specialist resources will be explored further in the next chapter in the context of looking at special areas of need.

THE WIDER SUPPORT NETWORK

In order to maintain this level and quality of care, there is one other vitally important resource necessary and that is the availability of personal support for the individual carer. Support of this kind must be seen as an essential ingredient to the resource facilities available and should be accepted as a normal and natural provision and not as a luxury or as something only needed for those who are weak or unable to cope, (Stoter, 1992).

The ability to draw on support from other members of the team, both from the multidisciplinary team and from one's own professional colleagues, is vital. It includes developing a caring attitude towards oneself in which it is recognised that, 'I am an individual of worth and importance needing to be valued as much as needing to take in nourishment day by day.' Taking care of oneself physically, mentally and spiritually, is a prerequisite for giving good total care to patients and families. A person whose own spiritual growth and development is undernourished will have little to share with others and their resources will quickly dry up when faced with the pressures of constant demand. The ability to value and respect the team with which one works and also to allow oneself to be valued and supported is essential in building up a healthy unified team stronger in their unity than as a group of isolated individuals. It is a fact well supported by research that a group identity has a quality over and above the sum of its individual members (Kretch *et al.* 1962; *see also Chapters 11–13*).

Those who hold positions of responsibility also need to recognise that they too require support if they are to be properly equipped in knowing how to give support to others. Part of this caring for the team is to give opportunity for more than just reporting. It is to explore the situation and to give opportunities for affirmation as well as developing knowledge and expertise. It may be that a less experienced member of the team has been caught up in a situation where the patient or family are requiring some explanation relating to matters of life and death which needed to be explored on the spot rather than evaded or postponed. Upon reflection that carer may feel he or she has dealt inadequately or wrongly with the situation and may come away torn by doubt and uncertainty, especially where there are no easy answers as so often happens with spiritual care. Such feelings of failure can cause the carer to avoid similar occasions in the future. There is a need to be able to follow-up that experience immediately with someone. Perhaps this will be another team member who is able to explore the experience as a learning situation giving affirmation and building on the positive achievement leaving the carer feeling more confident to cope the next time such an occasion arises.

The value of personal support

To give praise where it is due is equally important as giving a rebuke where necessary. A rebuke will be more effective if it is seen as coming from someone who can also give thanks and praise where they are due. Sadly, in the caring professions it seems that rebuke is often the only kind of communication passing from authority down the line. Peer support and support for the carers' families and friends can also help to give strength and stability and offer scope for natural refreshment and restoration away from the workplace.

For many staff the need is simply to be able to express fears, doubts and uncertainties in a safe environment in which the carer's professionalism will not be doubted because they share these universal emotions and reactions. It is essential to recognise that when putting on a uniform a person does not cease to be human but simply expresses a part of humanity from within a particular profession. Sensitivity and vulnerability are often looked upon as disadvantages, weaknesses and failures in those caring for others, when in reality they are qualities often found in the finest carers provided they are adequately supported and feel supported within themselves. Those who have come to terms with their own vulnerability and pain, and are not threatened or overwhelmed by them, are often a great resource to others as this experience helps their understanding of those who are suffering.

To be opening oneself to pain and suffering, to the sufferer's beliefs and to the patient's or family's search for meaning in life inevitably brings exposure to the carer's own beliefs. An essential part of resourcing for carers is to examine regularly their own values and beliefs and to identify what they feel to be important for themselves. Relatively speaking, the nature of a specific belief is of less importance in itself than an individual holding specific beliefs and knowing what they are. Unfortunately, because beliefs affect the ways in which we as individuals live our lives, there is a tendency for us to feel threatened and become more rigid in our views when our own beliefs are challenged. It takes great maturity and a confidence found by those who have thought through their own beliefs to a reasonable depth to allow the individual to stand comfortably with them.

It has been said that 'you don't really believe something until you can laugh at it and certainly until you can put it up for scrutiny without feeling threatened if someone else holds a contrary view'.

The final stage in that maturity is to be able to value the other person's beliefs even when they are quite contrary to our own. We need to be able to say, 'I disagree with what you say but I defend to the hilt your right to say it.'

Sadly in the field of personal belief there is often a strong desire for certainty. When not too sure of our own position, it may be difficult to allow anyone to put up a coherent alternative view as they may cause us to feel insecure and might undermine our own confidence. The open honest search for truth is always enriching even if at times it demands the death or adaptation of our former beliefs. Truth has many different facets depending on the perspective and maturity of the seeker. It is a bit like looking at the white light through a prism – you see different colours depending on where you stand – pure white light is always present but you don't always see it as such because the light is broken up into its seven different components. Truth also is 'a many splendoured thing' (Frances Thomson – *A Hymn of Love*).

> *'The atheist staring from his attic window is often nearer*
> *to God than the believer caught up in his own false image of God'*
>
> Martin Buber – *I and Thou*

This section has ranged widely over the topic of the carer as a major resource in the partnership and relationship essential to the provision of good spiritual care. The next section moves on to explore the patient's spiritual needs and response to suffering and care offered. This is inevitably a two-way process and needs to be viewed from the perspective of the patient, the carer and the interaction between them once the individual issues have been identified and explored.

QUESTION 1

Look up some of the recent literature on the use of alternative therapies. In what ways can they be of value to patients and clients? Assess some of the main current views for and against their use.

Key points

- No carer comes alone to offer spiritual care: there are resources through others in the team and through professional training.
- Carers do, however, bring their own unique range of professional skills and personal experience.
- Wider resources are available through the team. Their beliefs may be different but this is irrelevant if their skills are essential.
- Specific skills are available also within other professions, particularly the alternative therapies.
- Many patients today value the personal relationship offered with a therapist in these alternative approaches.
- Staff themselves need personal care, value and support to provide good quality care.

Section III

The patient's response

One of the prerequisites for good spiritual care, which we explored in Section II, was the importance of establishing a relationship of trust between the carer and the client or patient. Without such a relationship, much of the process of delivering spiritual care can be difficult. In addition to considering the carer's response to the need for care, we need to look at the response of the patient or client because the nature and quality of that response can influence greatly the kind of communication process and care which is appropriate.

The range of responses to the situation and to any approach from an individual carer will be very broad and vary according to the individual's maturity, life experience, culture, beliefs and values. There are certain patterns of response, however, which are common to many situations. These include the response of grief in cases of loss or the response of a person in shock and sudden trauma. This section will look at some of those general areas of response and trace some of the patterns which are recognisable. It will also consider the unpredictable nature of response and look at some of the relevant and appropriate aspects of spiritual care.

> *In order to arrive at what you do not know*
> *You must go by a way which is the way of ignorance*
> *In order to possess what you do not possess*
> *You must go by the way of dispossession.*
>
> TS Eliot – *East Coker, The Four Quartets*

CHAPTER 8

The emotional response to being a patient

THE SICK ROLE

It is important, first of all, to remember that the patient is responding continuously to a particular experience – that of 'being a patient'. The client is responding to the processes of investigation, treatment and recovery. There is also a personal and internal response to the way in which care is offered or to how the 'patient role' is presented by the carers, the family, visitors and colleagues. Responses may well be influenced by the nature of the treatment necessary, the patient's condition or by the side-effects of drugs given. These and many other factors will influence the way in which a particular person responds.

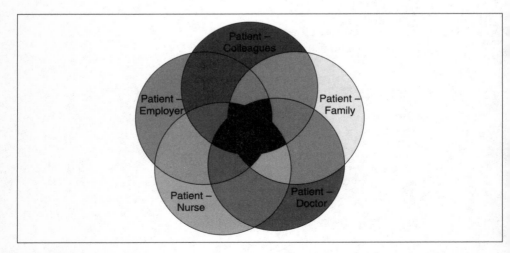

This diagram shows some of the different roles that a sick patient assumes, giving rise to different expectations and responses. Circles could be added to include friends, community, other carers etc.

An individual's internal response may be very different from that which is apparent on the surface. The patient is adjusting to what may be new situations and a range of different roles can be confusing. There are different responses to the family and relatives and to different professionals in ways thought to be acceptable to them and the patient may work hard to 'get it right' the first time. If they do not conform to patterns of response expected of them, the patient may fear being labelled uncooperative or difficult.

Theories and models: their use and abuse

There are several theoretical approaches which may help the reader to understand the nature of the 'sick role' and there are also models relating to patterns of response to grief and loss. Some of these are relevant here or will be referred to later in this section. (For those wishing to explore this area further, a useful discussion can be found in Cox, 1982, Chapter 8). In the last Chapter, we noted that these models should be recognised as devices which can help the carer to understand the processes taking place or can help in assessing what the patient's needs are and the most appropriate response. While they can be useful in preparing the carer, giving some idea of what kind of behaviour might be expected, it is important that they are not seen as stereotypes or models of anticipated behaviour as every person is an individual and will respond differently to any given situation.

EXAMPLES OF MODELS

One problem is found in Talcott Parsons' work (1951) presenting what is probably one of the best known approaches to studying the concept of the sick role and relationships between the patient and professionals. He describes ways in which society expects a sick person to behave and sets out the patient's rights and obligations by which he or she must seek recovery and follow proper medical advice. In return, the patient may expect sympathy and relief from normal responsibilities.

Parsons sees the roles of patient and doctor as reciprocal: the doctor having knowledge and skill and the patient being expected to trust the doctor while the relationship is guided by medical ethics. This approach places doctors and some other professionals in a very powerful and influential position. Parsons' theory assumes a basis of harmony and reciprocity, but other writers are critical of this approach (Bloor and Horobin, 1975).

Freisdon (1962) also sees a dilemma here and points out that patients and doctors enter into a relationship with considerable differences in their knowledge and experience of the situation and this can lead to a clash of perspectives, particularly if the patient tries to control the relationship.

A parallel example can often be seen at times when the patient's 'public persona' is poles away from the real 'persona'. This has two aspects: one being the patient's own perception of what is expected in 'normal behaviour' and response, and the other what society expects in terms of various groups such as the ward, the close-knit community and family etc. These may all project different roles of their own onto the patient. Individuals need to conform to accepted patterns to gain society's approval and so they follow what seems to be the anticipated norms.

Another theoretical approach worth comment here is seen in Goffman's work on Stigma (1963 and 1968). He discusses this concept as it relates to certain kinds of illness such as mental illness, handicap or physical disability. The stigma that society attaches to these and other illnesses may influence the kind of expectations the patient has concerning his care, whether he or she accepts the illness, refuses to acknowledge it, attempts to overcome and fight it or even to ignore it. Alternatively, it may be seen as a means of escape from responsibility.

EXERCISE 18
Working in your discussion group or with a colleague – bring some interesting examples you have experienced where a patient has presented 'public persona' which is remote from the "real" person they are. How do different professionals see or approach such a patient?

ROLES AND EXPECTATIONS

Thus it is clear that any of these different roles carry expectations which can create a facade, giving a false situation for communication. When truth or reality is not being acknowledged, it is difficult to engage in a relationship that allows for meeting the real spiritual needs. There is a complicated two-way process between the patient and carer, which requires recognition if both are to be tuned-in to one another. Carers need to be very conscious of this. It follows that any patient will be capable of any number of responses, which will vary according to their perception of their role and that of the person with them at any time, and also vary with their own attitudes to illness. The interaction may remain simply within the nature of 'role meeting role' in which the agenda is set by each person having a perceived view of their own needs and expectations and also of the other person. In our society, conformity wins approval and carers need to be sensitive to the effect this has on the patient's response.

THE NATURE OF THE RESPONSE

Some carers may unconsciously control the interaction by the projection of theories and models, responding to the expected needs which they have already decided are applicable to the patient's condition. The patient accepts this because of the need to retain the professional as an ally – they need to please the person who they see as having power over their life, their care and their process of recovery.

This can be illustrated by reference to processes with which carers may be most familiar, and which are often described in models. Many will be familiar with Kubler-Ross's description of the process of dying (1969). She describes the phases through which people pass as follows:
• Denial and isolation – allowing time for the collection of thoughts.

- Anger, rage and resentment are commonly expressed.
- Adjustment to guilt – there is often a bargaining process.
- Depression as it becomes evident denial is no longer possible.
- Acceptance bringing a measure of peace.

Carr (1982) says that while individuals' responses to the dying process show sufficient uniformity and similarity to other stressful situations to be credible, it is essential to recognise that individuals respond to stress situations in a personal way and with a particular self image. As each person is unique, classifications must be used with caution.

Sims (1988) summarises these two theoretical frameworks from different perspectives explaining responses to dying as follows: 'Responses to dying comprise a predictable sequential stress response to the process' or 'Responses to dying comprise a nonsequential stress response reflecting the individual's usual pattern of responding to stress'.

Dying is a personal experience

In other words, the event of dying is a highly personal experience and, at present, the evidence does not favour either of these approaches but the discussion is helpful for those trying to understand what is likely to happen. The carer, however, needs to retain a descriptive model of this kind as a guide, rather than imposing the process on the patient. Some patients will be able to raise issues and ask questions of the professional carers, while others may feel it is not proper or that they will be thought difficult, silly or childish if they ask. If the signals are not detected, the relationship does not progress. This may mean that the relationship only deals with surface needs and does not allow for meeting the deeper or demanding needs.

Often the earlier indicators of 'disease' are focused on immediate physical needs, discomfort, pain or an uncomfortable bed as being acceptable reasons for seeking attention. This is rather like the child's request 'Can I have a drink please?' when needing comfort. This opens up a need/response, question/answer equation, which is important when beginning to establish a relationship or trust but has the danger of establishing simply a problem solving response. As the indicators move into the aspects of personal life, family and friends, it is important that the carer avoids the simple problem-solving response and allows the exploration of the deeper underlying feelings. The practical problem solving response can help to establish the framework for spiritual care but needs to be used very sparingly when the deeper areas of feeling are explored.

The real heart of spiritual interaction is where feelings or emotions are allowed natural and appropriate expression alongside the clinical aspects of the patient's condition and needs. It is essential to respect that entry into deeper feelings by allowing the patient not only to respond to openness with openness but also to allow him to set the agenda and to have control over the communication process.

Finally, it must be underlined again that it is unwise to expect a particular emotional response but essential for carers to be ready to accept what is presented. If people are genuinely heard, their responses may take them in any direction allowing for expression as anger or rage, fear, doubt, guilt or anxiety, hopelessness, helplessness and despair. There may, at times, be a complete withdrawal into silence. This may be expressed verbally or physically, sometimes violently by tears or by clinging behaviour, or it may manifest itself internally, and there may be any combination of these. The essential ingredient here is the open accepting relationship in which the true feelings can be expressed by the patient or client, heard, valued and received by the carers.

QUESTION 1

Mrs P., who is aged 80 years, has grown up in a country village where the doctor was respected as someone to be treated with reverence and awe. She therefore responds politely to young registrars from that perspective. The nurses and physiotherapists, however, have a very different impression of a garrulous and cantankerous patient who tells each one of them a different story. Discuss some of the problems arising and suggest ways of overcoming these.

QUESTION 2

Describe a model you are familiar with and then discuss a situation where you have found it a useful guide to practice. How has it helped or hindered you?

Key points

- The patient's response, while differing from the carer's, needs to be seen always in the context of the relationship
- The sick role brings for the patient a whole host of new and bewildering roles and relationships
- The new roles involve a range of people and experiences
- Theories and models help in understanding the processes of response, but need to be applied cautiously in individual situations
- One example given – the response to dying which is a highly personal experience

The patient's response to suffering, pain and loss

*These people are the hollowed bamboo through which
the life giving water flows, the reed pipe on which the
musician plays his song.*

Sheila Cassidy – *Good Friday People*

This Chapter looks at the patient's response to some specific aspects of suffering related to illness, trauma or injury. Suffering is a very complex process and, as responses can be affected by a wide range of influences, the nature of the response is also complex and varies between different situations. When looking at some of the specific areas of suffering, it is apparent that there are some common elements and there is a great deal of interaction between the various responses. For example, the severity of pain may well be affected by the individual's state of tension or relaxation or by the level of fear or confidence experienced. A person who is cold responds differently from one who is warm and comfortable. Hence there is the need to view the person as a whole rather than a series of isolated stages.

An individual who is suffering, whatever the cause, responds to that suffering with his total being. A range of feelings will be experienced and these may be expressed by an equally wide range of behaviour patterns, most of which can be recognised as normal expected responses – part of the normal process of responding to illness, injury, recovery or loss. Sometimes the process of response is delayed for some reason, however, resulting in an abnormally prolonged period of depression, which needs expert professional care (Parkes, 1972).

As already indicated, it is not easy to separate and classify the various causes of suffering and specific responses as the whole subject is interwoven and complex. Pain may be physical, emotional or social. It may be equally intense whatever the cause and it is indicative of some kind of personal spiritual suffering. Emotional suffering is strongly evident after shock, bereavement or loss arising from a variety of reasons. As pain is a common element in most forms of suffering or loss, responses to pain or suffering will be considered first and then we will look at the response to specific kinds of loss, which is a factor in some way in most kinds of suffering. This Chapter concludes with looking at grief patterns and bereavement related to the loss of an individual who has been close to the bereaved person.

RESPONSE TO PAIN AND SUFFERING

Everyone experiences pain of some kind at different times in their lives and all have developed responses that are related to earlier experiences in life in the home, family or school. For example, in our own culture, a degree of stoicism is rewarded by social approval – children may be rewarded in some way if they do not cry when grazing their knees or visiting the dentist. A 'stiff upper lip' response is generally commended as being a sign of courage. To minimise the level of pain is seen to be acceptable if only to make things easier for family, friends or staff to care for them. For this reason, it is a response given much support. There are cultures where it is expected that pain will be expressed openly in tears and words. This is sometimes noticeable during birth of a child despite an effective epidural injection.

> 'There is a cold fear in a time of tribulation,
> A time of the olive press, the wine press,
> The crushing grapes
> And no guarantee of a good vintage
> Jim Cotter – *Healing – More or Less.*

Factors influencing pain

A number of factors influence the severity of pain experienced and therefore the kind of response evoked. Attitudes can be affected by expectations that pain will be relieved or perhaps, more importantly, will not be relieved. Hence, there is the need for accurate assessment and effective pain relief, which gives a powerful message to the patient and often leads to lower levels of analgesia being required. In addition, anxiety levels decrease as levels of confidence increase. Expectations also play a large part in childbirth where a distressing experience with a first delivery can lead to expectations of a repeat performance and can increase apprehension and anxiety for future births.

Studies concerning levels of pain have concluded that individual people have different pain thresholds. It is accepted that some individuals experience pain more intensely than others and that this will vary at different times and with different situations. The interdependence between the physical and psychological cause of pain makes it important that any assessment should include accurate measurement and consideration of the individual's total pain responses: the intensity of pain, emotional physical, social and spiritual response should be measured. Attention to response in any one of these areas can raise the pain threshold and give some relief, (Corovan, 1991). Each individual has different thresholds for different kinds of pain. For example, a person with a high tolerance of physical pain may have a low tolerance with regard to loss of dignity, as with incontinence, or to the pain of loss of a much loved relative.

Links with anxiety and past experiences

There is a need for a proper diagnosis and a balance between consideration of the different causes of pain. To simply treat the physical pain is to ignore the wider aspects of suffering and does the patient a disservice. There is clearly a link with anxiety arising from any aspect of the situation – one only has to tense up the muscles when sitting in an uncomfortable chair to discover how quickly it becomes painful and appreciate how tension can increase pain. Wherever there is an attempt to suppress pain and suffering, that in itself should be seen as a signal indicating distress. Feeling alone and isolated is also likely to exacerbate pain, whereas feeling cared for and comfortable can have the opposite effect.

For many people, this kind of response links back with childhood situations and bad experiences early in life, for example, when a frightened or hurt baby or child needed to be held to relieve the pain. This is where staying with a patient going through a painful experience and sharing their feelings, particularly linking in with their feelings through touch, can bring some aspect of relief. Physical manifestations of pain can be recognised in the ways in which patients sit, lie or hold themselves when there is an obvious element of tension or reluctance to change position. They are often reluctant to complain verbally for fear of being thought childish, silly or a nuisance. Once able to share the worst of the situation, relaxation may begin and the patient begins to look more comfortable as being listened to is, in itself, therapeutic. One particular response to pain and suffering which brings relief to some is to create a secondary area of pain to take the mind off the original cause. This may take the form of head-banging, inflicting self wounds or creating a confrontation which allows for pain to be expressed and transferred to the family or staff.

EXERCISE 19
Conside how your family relationships affect your personal responses to suffering, pain and loss. (This is a personal exercise for your own record.)

THE RESPONSE TO LOSS

`We must learn to regard people less in the light of what
they do or omit to do, but more in the light of what they suffer'
Dietrich Bonhoeffer (source unknown)

It is clear that responses to pain and suffering overlap. They are also interwoven with the response to loss and bereavement. There is a considerable element of loss involved with many aspects of life including sickness, injury, redundancy from work, failure or ageing. Most suffering is related to loss of one kind or another and just being a patient in hospital can bring a threatening loss of liberty and freedom by separation from family, friends, familiar surroundings, work and social life.

Bereavement associated with loss of a person is not the only kind of bereavement but, as it is such a major event at some time in life for most people, it merits separate attention, which is given later in this book. Response patterns associated with any form of loss, however, are similar and normal grief encompasses a wide range of feelings and behaviour. Such feelings include anger, guilt, self-reproach, anxiety, helplessness, rage, fatigue, numbness, shock and disbelief. Physical manifestations may include general symptoms of fear, sweating, trembling, nausea, tight throat and chest, dry mouth, and general weakness and fatigue. There may be disturbances in sleeping and eating patterns, crying, overactivity and, over a period of time, depression and withdrawal. The stages in behaviour patterns have been described by many writers (references to these are found in Chapter 8 where the value of these models was discussed). Descriptions are generally on similar lines including:

- Shock and denial, with the initial impact of loss.
- The process of developing awareness, anger and bargaining.
- Finally, resolution and acceptance.

(Speck, 1978; Cook and Phillips, 1988; Parkes, 1975).

In its broadest sense, loss means separation from something which has been an integral part of the person's being (Cook and Phillips, 1988) and it inevitably involves a period of change and adjustment. To understand the impact of loss and associated behaviour, it is helpful to remind ourselves of the influences of childhood experiences relating to the process of bonding and the importance of attachment in providing secure and safe relationships (Bowlby, 1977; Worden 1983). When the attachment figure is threatened, the response is one of intense anxiety and the closer the attachment, the more powerful are the emotions experienced.

The wide range of different influences and experiences makes the effects of loss and the response to it very variable. Effects of loss depend on factors such as time of life, the situation in relation to other events, the support of family and friends, personality, cultural differences and the practical implications for work, financial security or career prospects.

We only have to look at the range of situations involving some aspect of loss and to register the wide variations of response which may be encountered to see the enormous challenge that faces the carer in this field .

EXERCISE 20

Now think about someone you know who has recently experienced some kind of loss. How did that person respond? Look at this in a group discussion and identify responses that occur most often. Which are the responses that are difficult to observe?

SUDDEN LOSS

In its widest form this is the most dramatic and thus most easily recognised form of loss. It brings with it sudden curtailment of liberty if the individual is detained in hospital. It may be caused by accident, unexpected illness or surgical treatment or there may be a major loss of limb or serious disfigurement caused by injury. This obviously causes severe shock with the accompanying responses of disbelief, denial, anger and rage. Less easily recognised is the potential loss involved in such sudden trauma and this is an area of loss which is a major challenge in a range of situations and is often overlooked (Wright, 1991).

POTENTIAL LOSS

Incidents like those just mentioned bring with them a host of possibilities and threatening situations, which can give rise to anxiety and uncertainty so adding to the tensions created by the immediate shock. There is the disorientating effect of separation from family and work for a while, which brings with it the threat of loss of job, financial loss and possible career and relationship limitations. This anxiety often presents in a panic reaction and restlessness as the victim searches for reassurance and new securities.

The threat of potential loss is also present in many cases of disability, long-term illness or progressive disease where the outcome and extent of the ultimate loss are not yet fully apparent. Patients often find it difficult to face possibilities and realities here and so present defence or distancing mechanisms or refuse to accept growing limitations or make necessary adjustments. Incidentally, this is also a common response in normal ageing processes where individuals find it hard to accept the limitations of physical ageing and refuse to make allowances for a changing capability or loss of ability. This response is often manifest in extreme bouts of frustration, irritability and later by depression as reality begins to dawn, and may indirectly cause accidents or injury. For the ageing, there is loss of independence, for example: they can no longer do their own decorating or gardening; they may no longer be able to live alone and so have to give up the home; they may have to accept a wheelchair for mobility; or they may have to accept the child or children in a reversed power role where the parent is now dependent upon the child.

The threat of potential loss is also an area where false hopes are often expressed such as 'perhaps the doctor might be wrong' or 'nature is a wonderful healer' or 'miracles do happen'. There is an atmosphere of unreal false optimism as people refuse, or are unable at that time, to face the facts. Family and friends or professionals can knowingly encourage this as it makes communication less threatening if the patient is talking of recovery and not of death or disablement.

Example
Sometimes a careless phrase may unwittingly encourage false hopes. For example, the parents of a baby born with major complex heart problems were seen by a doctor who explained carefully and clearly the nature of the problem and said at least four times, 'Expect your baby to die tonight'. In response to the question, 'But can't you do anything?' he replied, 'No – nothing'. When asked, 'Are you sure?', he replied, 'Yes,' and then unfortunately, as he admitted later, out of a feeling of helplessness and a desire to do something for them he added, 'Should she survive the night, which I doubt, I will take some blood tests and X rays tomorrow.' When the doctor left the

room, the mother turned to the father and said, 'I'm so relieved – he can help our baby after all'. Within a few minutes the baby was dead.

Other areas of threat from potential loss face those who are partially sighted or suffering from loss of hearing – the latter is an instance where people postpone the use of a hearing aid for longer than necessary as they find difficulty in accepting deafness.

LOSS OF BODY IMAGE

This is also an aspect of loss which often suffers from lack of recognition. Such loss may be caused by amputation or by major surgery with resulting disfigurement, which can cause considerable distress and feelings of bereavement. Presentation of an acceptable public face is important to many people as is evident by the time spent in choice of dress, use of beauty aids, cosmetics, deodorants, etc. The body image is powerfully tied up with this public presentation, which, if altered, damaged or scarred by injury or treatment, may be distressing and sometimes unacceptable to those around. The individual may lose worth in the eyes of others as well as in their own eyes. Other instances of damaged body image occur where permanent changes occur to normal function. For example, many patients find difficulty accepting a stoma and its permanence and often need help with this.

Self-image is very much linked to 'what I do rather than who I am' and when a person feels he or she is seen as unable to contribute effectively, this may lead to a loss of self worth. Thus, something like an amputation can have far-reaching effects on an individual's perception of their ability to progress in their chosen career or to continue their social activities. Their perception is often one of being incomplete: indeed, mobility and dexterity can be affected in a way that makes them feel unacceptable to others and also to themselves.

SOME MORE COMPLEX ASPECTS OF LOSS

The discussion so far shows that some aspects of loss are clearly apparent to the observer, while others are much less tangible and therefore their influence, in terms of the patient's response, may pass unrecognised. For example, a physical disability or the loss of a limb or a faculty such as sight is very clear to any casual observer. What is often more obscure is the associated loss of mobility causing dependency. This has long-term implications concerning limitations of independence and alterations in lifestyle. There may be related loss or limitation of career prospects, with consequent changes in income and lifestyle. These could have major effects on someone who has led an active physical life, for example, an athlete or a building labourer. Such loss has far-reaching effects on family relationships and lifestyle, which can evoke a more devastating response than the original deprivation itself. (This will be explored further when looking at the response of adaptation in Chapter 10.)

LOSS OF COMMUNICATION

Loss of communication may be caused by loss of speech or hearing. Either way it is a very significant aspect of loss associated with certain illnesses – particularly stroke, forms of coma or even during unconsciousness. This can be particularly frustrating, humiliating and distressing, especially where the patient is fully aware of what is going on and is unable to respond or to express their desperation. It is always important for the carer to remember that even where verbal communication is impaired, the individual may still hear and understand what is being said. Thus, other methods of communicating need to be explored.

Loss of habit is another element which is often underestimated in this kind of situation. We are very much creatures of habit in our daily lifestyle. For example, the way in which we start the day usually follows a particular pattern or routine. The way in which we wash, shower, bath, brush our teeth, shave, apply make-up or dress follows the same pattern day after day. Sequence of any kind brings a sense of order and normality and a comfortable sense of control in managing the affairs of everyday life. Any disruption of such routine can bring about feelings of disorientation and uncertainty. This is particularly evident in bereavement where loss of a relationship is concerned.

Loss of control is perhaps one of the most powerful elements in almost every situation of loss. It is natural to want to be in control of one's own life – teenagers prefer to take control of their lives from their parents. Consequently, to be in a position where what is most important is beyond the person's control, for example in life-and-death situations, thus has a major impact. The patient may be experiencing new and strong feelings for the first time and entering into a totally unfamiliar territory where he or she feels bewildered, disorientated and uncertain about how to respond. It is likely that there will be evidence of the responses previously mentioned. These could include shock and total denial, anger, rage and withdrawal from the situation until the sufferer is able to find new responses with the discovery of other coping mechanisms.

There are also aspects of loss associated with changes in circumstances, such as redundancy, retirement, loss of status or loss of possessions. These are perhaps less tangible and therefore responses may not be recognised and the often dramatic changes in behaviour patterns may be misunderstood. Each of these is a bereavement in itself and all the related responses may follow (Cook and Phillips, 1988).

VARIATIONS IN RESPONSE

Most people have at some time or another to stand alone
to suffer, and their final shape is determined by their response
to their probation. They emerge either slaves of circumstance
or in some sense captains of their souls.

Charles G Raven – *A Wanderer's Way*

Just as the range of response to all these aspects of loss varies considerably, so the pace of response can be affected by pressure from family or professionals. There may be pressures to come to terms with the loss, or accept and move ahead too quickly, which can increase feelings of inadequacy. Alternatively, the converse may be present when there is too much 'support' or over-protection, which can encourage excessive dependency. The process of coming to terms with loss is a very personal one and helping someone in this journey is a delicate process. It is important that the individual is not held back by too much optimism or pushed ahead too quickly when what they need is someone to walk with them at their own pace.

Specific beliefs born of the culture in which an individual has been nurtured will influence the way in which an experience is evaluated and will effect the nature of the response. Any experience of pain or loss, here and now, is related to the image of who and what a person has been in the past. It is affected by the extent to which they saw themselves as a relatively fit person with all the capacity to move forward in life and control their own destiny. Pain is the pain of here and now, but it is related to the person and situation lost and longed for – the person they once were and who can no longer be expressed in the same way.

Spiritual care relating to these responses

Thus with any experience of loss, there is a powerful backward focus to be recognised in the memory of what has been done, achieved, accepted as normal and taken for granted but now there is a desperate pain for what can no longer be. Spiritual care is basically about getting to know the person cared for in the here and now, coming to know as much as possible about the person, listening and walking alongside in the journey of life and aiding in the process of coming to terms with loss and its consequences.

Some will respond by complete hopelessness and despair, while others develop determination, courage and faith in recovery or adaptation and find a new purpose for living. There are a few unusual individuals who, like Simon Weston of the Falklands fame, can turn their loss into a personal triumph and develop a new identity through their misfortune.

QUESTION 1
Consider a patient you have recently cared for who has experienced real physical or emotional pain. Describe some particular responses and compare these with similar situations you have met. Why do individual responses differ?

QUESTION 2
Consider the situation of three different individuals who have recently experienced a severe loss of some kind:
(a) Jane who is 39 years old, happily married with three teenage children and has just had a mastectomy.
(b) Michael who is 44 years old and is a skilled craftsman in a manufacturing industry. He has recently had his right arm amputated following an accident.

(c) Jamie who is 10 years old and has recently lost his sight following an accident. Discuss the nature of the response for each of these and identify some of the spiritual needs to be met.

❀

Key points

- There are common elements in most responses to pain and suffering.
- The intensity or nature of the pain will influence the particular response.
- Levels of pain are affected by anxiety, fear and past experience.
- Levels of pain are affected by communications of family, friends and professionals.
- Loss involves a period of change and adjustment.
- The nature of the loss needs to be identified to understand the responses.
- Loss is a bereavement.

Responding to particular aspects of suffering – why me?

Suffering is suffering, there's no argument about that.
It hurts. It is painful.

Herman Hesse

In essence, bereavement does not differ from any other kind of loss. The overall reactions and responses follow similar patterns. It is the depth and length of the reaction and response that is important and this is related to the loss of a significant person who, to state the obvious, is never coming back. Here, there is loss of a relationship and of normal habits of daily living which have evolved over the years. It is obvious that loss of habit is a general feature of any form of loss but it is perhaps more potent where a personal relationship is concerned.

LOSS OF HABIT

Loss of habit is, by definition, a powerful element in bereavement as habits of a lifetime will have been destroyed. This is so even in situations where, to the outside observer, relationships have been negative, dominant or submissive. A hen-pecked partner or the hen-pecking partner may miss the personality of the other as the habitual complementary personality has gone, so removing a very large and important aspect of daily interaction.

It may be difficult, for example, to go to the pub or cinema alone when the habit has been to go as a couple. This can be difficult to understand for the person who is used to doing so alone or used to gathering a group friends together for such visits. So the habit element is often ignored or very underestimated as a feature of loss. Emotionally, it is a demanding experience to reassess all aspects of living and to build in new habits.

Some people respond to bereavement by a process of blocking or repressing their feelings. This is sometimes a response created for them by the inappropriate responses of others that make it difficult for them to express their feelings freely. Sometimes families, friends or professional staff can unwittingly encourage a person to turn in upon themselves by projecting a coping image that is not felt, so making them feel separate and isolated from the world. A feeling of not being understood can lead to bitterness and a withdrawal from people and social interaction. This is where professional staff have an important role to play to ensure that the individual is free to respond in an appropriate way to the loss so that he or she can express feelings and explore the reality of the situation.

LOSS OF RELATIONSHIP THROUGH BEREAVEMENT

Loss of a parent

The nature of a response to the loss of a close relationship will vary according to place in the family group. Loss of a parent can be particularly devastating but, with an aged parent this is a natural expectation built into most people's thinking about parents. Most of us live as if that event will never happen and yet, when it does happen, it has a normality about it as being part of the normal course of events, particularly when the parent has reached a great age.

This is, however, the loss of a key relationship. There is a greater dependency on parents early in life, but it is a relationship that breeds certain habits that will change over a lifetime as the dependency roles are interchanged. Roles are reversed when the child grows up and becomes a parent in their own right. Their own parent eventually becomes dependent on them for support, while the son or daughter takes over more responsibility and care. A threatening dimension is that the bereaved individuals are reminded that they themselves are now the senior generation. This is a natural reminder for everyone of mortality and of the inevitability of eventual death for all of us.

The loss of a parent can have devastating and long-term effects for a young child, which vary according to the child's age, quality of the relationship and family life. The immediate response of the child who is shocked and bewildered may be one of detachment and withdrawal at first. This can be associated with other signs of regressive behaviour, such as refusal to eat or speak, constant crying, eneuresis, violence or general detachment. The situation may be complicated by the remaining parent being devastated and unable to communicate or being unaware of the child's needs, thinking a young child does not understand (Raphael, 1985; Cook and Phillips, 1988).

Unfortunately it is often thought that if a child is not allowed to participate in the events surrounding the death, such as the funeral, then the child will not grieve. So at the time of the death and funeral, friends and other relatives often take the child away to give him or her 'treats'. The loss of a parent is thus compounded by the child being separated from the remaining parent who is the natural source of love and comfort. This may lead to anger and resentment in the long term and/or a feeling of not being of any importance. It may even make the child feel that he or she is being punished.

Bereavement is a very complex situation for a young child and needs specialist care. An element of loss may be inherent in many forms of parental deprivation or separation causing severe emotional disturbances for the child in later years. (For more detailed reading see: Bowlby, 1969; Kelner Pringle, 1975; Winnacott, 1964.)

Example

Lucy was 2 years old when her grandmother died after a short illness. Lucy had been taken to visit her grandmother daily and, because the grandmother was blind, she had held on to Lucy's hand firmly as they enjoyed many games together. A strong bond had developed between the two.

Lucy was protected carefully from all knowledge of activities surrounding the death and funeral. She constantly asked for Grandma and was told the old lady was 'resting' and 'had a headache'. After a few weeks her grief was ignored and her bewilderment was increased on hearing Grandma 'has gone away to be with Jesus' and later 'No, she isn't coming back'. No further details were given. She was vaguely aware of the black clothes, the hushed voices and the tearfulness of those around her and gradually began to feel she must be to blame because 'she had been too much for Grandma'. The child became withdrawn and lost her sparkle. Lucy grew up to be a lonely and detached child and 20 years on she developed an anxiety state following illness. Therapy revealed a loss of memory during the period in which she was 2–5 years old, a terror of separation from friends and family and severe panics related to illness. Gradually, as the story was unravelled, these symptoms began to subside and she became a much happier person, more able to trust and relate to friends, and later to have a successful professional career.

EXERCISE 20

Consider the above example and suggest some of ways in which Lucy might have been helped with the loss of her grandmother. What were some of the key factors in her family's approach that led to the later difficulties?

The loss of a spouse

> *A man's dying is more the survivor's affair than his own.*
> Thomas Mann (1875–1955).

The loss of a spouse is the loss of a person with whom the deepest revelations of self have been made and wherein lies the deepest knowledge and acceptance of the 'spiritual person'. This inevitably leaves the survivor alone and lonely. It does not matter how many people visit or the way in which they visit, the core relationship has gone and it is hard, particularly in the early days, for the partner to cope or to find the motivation to live. Many people live through life hoping that they will be the first to die and in that expectation have grown used to believing that separation will not happen to them.

When the death of the spouse or partner happens it is particularly powerful if the death is sudden or unexpected. Where illness has intervened, there will have been a period of time in which the lifestyle has changed to accommodate the illness and so some preparation may have taken place. With sudden death, however, there is no time for adaptation.

This relationship has a very special significance in that it is a personal relationship which has been chosen whereas with blood relations there is no choice. Spouses are people who have so impressed the heart and mind of the other person and *vice versa* that the two are committed to each other. If the relationship has been close, strong bonds are formed and strengthened through living together and in sharing the traumas of family life. If there are children, they present a challenge in bringing them up and establishing their lives and families.

There is thus a major area of commitment and mutual dependence which is equal to the quality of the relationship wherein the most important habits have been established together. Two individuals have come together with their own habits of a lifetime, which have been combined and grown into the habits of a marriage. This has happened through a process which has sometimes been a most costly compromise of habits, beliefs and actions.

THE LOSS OF A CHILD

The death of a child, whatever the age, is a particularly powerful loss as it goes against the natural order of things. It is expected that children bury parents and not the other way round. Most professionals also relate strongly to the powerful impact of the death of a child and its effect on themselves, the parents and other members of the family (Thomas, 1990).

The serious illness and death of a child or young person challenges the accepted role of parents to be able to provide for the needs of their children; to put right things that go wrong; to give security and to see them through into adulthood; or to provide care for the child who is the product of their love and who has had a strong level of dependence upon them for succour and nurture.

There are two kinds of loss to be considered here. First, there is the potential sense of loss which arises when parents are facing the news that their child is likely to die in the not too distant future. Second, there is the kind of loss involved with a sudden unexpected death. Although there are common elements in the responses to both types of loss, there are also particular reactions to the two different situations.

The threat of potential loss

When faced with the potential death of a child, parents often feel completely powerless. There is a strong sense of frustration and failure over their inability to carry out the parental role of care which anticipates the normal development of a healthy child through teenage years into adulthood. The challenge of potential loss, however, is different: it is debilitating and exhausting. It not only involves watching the child die but also trying to be available with loving support and practical help to maintain a quality of life. Supporting the rest of the family at the same time is an additonal pressure.

This deeply challenges any parent's humanity as there are feelings that the situation is all so unfair: that this is happening to a child who has not had a chance to live and who is being cut off from his or her potential life. These feelings may be exacerbated by comments from distressed grandparents or other older family members and friends who will say 'Why is it not me? I've had my life'. Parents themselves often feel they would willingly change places with their child if they could, feeling that a child should not have to face this.

These are powerful and conflicting emotions complicated by a desire to run away from the threat of what lies ahead, yet never moving from the bedside so that they can give all the care possible and do everything for the child themselves. There are mixed feelings of love, hurt, compassion and fear juxtaposed with feelings of immense anger and frustration governed by the sense of failure and powerlessness.

The natural parental feelings are to love the child, to want the best under any circumstances and to give and receive as much as possible. First reactions are a bit like falling in love in the early days when a couple just want to be together all the time. As time passes, they begin to reach a stage where love has deepened and others are drawn into the circle from outside and assume an important place in their activities. So when facing such a situation, parents tend to focus on their own child to the exclusion of other members of the family. They find it hard to accept even necessary care, which may appear at times to interfere with their desire to hold on to that relationship.

There is indeed a deep suffering in such love bringing pain beyond description. However much love is given, there is always a desire to give more. The prospect of sharing love is made more poignant by the knowledge that the relationship will come to an end before long and then such sharing will no longer be possible.

This inevitably brings with it a sense of anger and frustration beyond description in its intensity. As they anticipate the love that was to be which cannot be offered for much longer, they foresee only desolation. They almost want to force the child to get well and to find a reason for him to live longer. This can be a very powerful pressure on the professional carers who are well aware of their own limitations in the face of impending death, and of their inability to deliver what the parents most desire.

The effects of strong emotions

The parents' feelings of anger may also be directed towards themselves in relation to feelings of inadequacy and failure when their child is not going to live. Parents' anger towards themselves may be caused by them sensing that they feel unreasonably angry towards friends, relatives and carers. This anger can be fuelled by feeling that the situation is out of control.

The expression of such deep emotions is very tiring and brings with it both physical and mental exhaustion. On one hand, parents want oblivion from it all and on the other, they want the strength to carry on. Such exhaustion also brings with it a weakening of the immune system making them more susceptible to colds and viral infections.

The effects on the family

This exhaustion also finds its way into relationships with siblings and other members of the family and perhaps, at its worst, threatens relationships with the other children, or between the spouses or partners. Strong roles can develop: the mother may spend most of her time with the sick child while the father tries to balance work and organisation of the siblings; others might help them by collecting children from school. This brings a new dimension into the marriage relationship with altered responsibilities between the parents which affect the nature of their emotional responses to each other and to the siblings.

At times each parent may long for the death to come and then they will project feelings of guilt and anger towards themselves. The siblings who may be upset and frightened by what is happening to the brother or sister may find it difficult to get attention and show some of the feelings already described (see page ???). Such attention-seeking behaviour is often interpreted as naughtiness by the parents and their responses can lead to a child believing that the dying child is more important. The child might feel that the parents would rather he or she was dying instead of the sibling.

The death of a child is a very particular kind of loss for it is separation from part of oneself. It is the only relationship where another person has issued from oneself. So it is loss of oneself physically, emotionally and spiritually in terms of the existing bond and also the dependency of the child on those who have created him.

Part of the human quest for immortality lies in people's ability to reproduce and see themselves in their offspring with perpetuation of the family name. Death of a child deals a severe blow to that hope. Response is very far reaching and particularly so where the child is the creation of an especially loving relationship.

The sudden death of a child

In the event of sudden death, much of the response will mirror that already described above, but there is the added dimension that there has been no prior warning of death or any opportunity to prepare for that death in any sense. It is literally a devastating blow in which the whole structure of the family is shattered. The level of shock experienced will normally be considerable with very violent emotions of anger and rage directed right across the family. For the individuals most closely concerned, this anger is also directed inwards upon themselves in some circumstances (Raphael, 1985).

This is particularly true in the case of road accidents, drowning accidents, or accidents in the home or playground. In such cases, it is often seen that the accident could have been avoided and all the 'if onlys' arise: 'If only I had been there'; 'If only I had warned her'; 'If only he had listened to me'; or 'If she had done her job properly', and so on. This all leads to emotions expressing reproach, regret, anger and guilt – the effects of which may last for many years to come. Such devastating shock frequently brings with it a powerful sense of isolation followed by a retreat into oneself and a physical coldness, which may create a barrier difficult to penetrate. The death of a young adult can be equally traumatic for the parents with the additional dimension of the loss of a developed relationship with a young person in whom they have invested much love, hope and plans for the future.

Guilt and self blame are particularly powerful in this kind of death. Sometimes a seemingly logical picture has been built up, which can only be unravelled by seeing it in context.

EXAMPLE

I saw the parents of a 15-year-old boy in ITU. The boy had asked his father to take him by car to get something from a shop. His father told him to take his bike and get it himself. The boy rode his bike over a pedestrian crossing when the lights were against him and was knocked down. The father blamed himself and the mother blamed the father – tension levels ran high. It eventually turned out, of course, that this had happened many times before without incident. This realisation in time helped to lower the tensions and restore support.

MISCARRIAGE AND STILLBIRTH

The patient's response to childbirth

It is clear that much of the care in the obstetric department is concerned with providing a service for fit and healthy women giving birth to normal healthy babies. Childbirth is a powerful spiritual experience in that it involves the whole of each person who participates and parents and staff too. At a deeper level, it engages emotions, hopes, expectations and indeed fears and apprehensions. The more spiritually aware the family is, the more they will be aware of the responsibilities, challenges and demands of parenthood and the more they will want to approach these issues seriously. In the majority of cases, the outcomes for all concerned, and thus spiritual care, takes the form of encouragement along the way and sharing in the family's rejoicing and hopes for the future.

Where abnormality of the foetus is diagnosed, a difficult decision on whether or not to have a termination has to be assessed. This is a difficult ethical area giving rise to strong anxieties. Sometimes differences of opinion may arise between parents or in the wider family. Later in this book we refer to this and other issues but here we must recognise that the loss of a baby usually involves very powerful responses and distress. Expecting the birth of a child, assuming it is a wanted child, is a time of looking forward, anticipation, exploration of hopes and a time of dreams. For a couple wanting a family or an addition to their family, this pregnancy is a time of planning and preparation for a child with all its needs. It is a time of hope and anticipation of having a fit and healthy child who will perhaps mirror themselves in looks, attitude and integrity.

The parents are able to fantasise by looking into the future and they anticipate not only the birth but actually holding the baby. They can visualise the baby's features and watching it grow up. They imagine the child in a variety of situations such as riding a bike, kicking a ball, climbing a tree, going to school and watching its every moment of growth. There may be dreams of growing up:

'Who will he be like?'; 'Who will she marry?'; 'Will I have grandchildren?'.

All of these big hopes can suddenly be dashed to pieces in a moment of time when the child is stillborn or when a miscarriage occurs.

Miscarriage, stillbirth or infant death

As Hopper reminds us, the parents are suddenly faced with the 'profound combination of childbirth and death together' – two equally strong, if contrasting, emotions (Hopper, 1991). Many people underestimate the depth of an experience in which death and birth are in such close proximity. They fall into the trap of believing the grief cannot be as great because the child has not lived, but it has actually been part of the family since conception was known to the parents. The love for that child has already begun as the natural extension of the love the couple have for each other is deepened by the anticipation and preparation of the birth.

The loss is very powerful and contains a strong sense of unfairness that the baby has had no chance to live a life. This sense can be reinforced when the baby is seen, held and grieved for. The levels of pain and devastation are extremely high as hopes and expectations have been dashed by stillbirth or miscarriage. The couple are transported from hope to devastation in a short space of time. The intensity of emotional response is not related to gestational age, so the levels of pain and grief for miscarriage are no less than those for stillborn babies or those that die after a period of independent life (Pepper and Knapp, 1980).

The child handicapped from birth

The birth of a handicapped child also triggers powerful feelings of loss. It is a big challenge to come to terms with a child who was expected to be strong, fit and healthy, being born handicapped.

Guilt is a strong emotion here indeed the initial response may often be one of rejection of the child. It may be that the parents cannot bear to look at the child as it is because it becomes so threatening and devastating to them. This does not necessarily mean they will be unable to cope with the child or give it love later when needed. The process of adjusting completely to realistic levels may well become difficult, particularly where the parents and others in the family are high achievers.

THE CHILD'S RESPONSE TO ILLNESS AND DEATH

The loss of a parent in particular has already been mentioned briefly early in this Chapter. With children involved in any way with an experience of illness or death, the effects are likely to be very complex. These effects will vary with the age and developmental stage of the child, as well as with the nature of the relationship with the person who has died (Raphael, 1985). Some adults find it difficult to understand that many children are aware of the implications and seriousness of illness and approaching death. It is also a commonly held belief that by avoiding the subject and denying any opportunity for discussing the situation, the child will remain in ignorance.

Many people who have experience of working with seriously or terminally ill children have observed that they are often quick to understand the seriousness of the situation and the possibility of death. Where support is given, it enables the sharing of information together with loving care and support. Children are frequently enabled to come to terms with their own death. Many families and professional staff will bear testimony that children have been able to help others around them to come to terms with impending death.

Avoiding the situation also misses the point that, for a sick child, illness affects the whole of his person and brings obvious limitations to many everyday activities. Illness frequently brings discomfort and pain together with the need for treatments which are themselves unpleasant. The child's mind, as is the case with the adult mind, is challenged and puzzled by what is happening in the illness and can experience a wide range of emotions and responses to the illness. To deny the opportunity for these to be expressed and responded to creates a deep level of isolation and may lead to anxiety, fear and subsequent regression.

Illness threatens the basic security of well being and the ability to satisfy the basic need to be secure and understood and to be allowed to express emotions that are there. There is a need to be respected as a human being, to be accepted and listened to and to come to terms with various losses involved in the particular illness. In some children, the illness may involve considerable debility, for example, in those with a chronic condition like cystic disease, which has a pattern likely to be increasingly disabling. Denial of access to information needed or avoidance of truth may simply reinforce any latent fears the child may have.

One difficulty adults experience when working with children is that the children can change mood or direction much more quickly than adults. At one moment they are talking with high emotion about the illness and death, and the next moment they switch to something light such as their favourite TV programme, video or music. This may in some way be related to the limited attention span that most children have. In addition to the behavioural changes already noted earlier in this Chapter, children often suffer from feelings of guilt, blaming themselves for what has happened, and fearing some pending punishment (Cook and Phillips, 1988). They may retreat into ritualistic or symbolic activities, which may persist unnoticed and unresolved until later years when skilled help may be needed to unravel the origins of depression or other forms of latent grief.

SIBLINGS: THEIR RESPONSE TO THE ILLNESS OF ANOTHER CHILD IN THE FAMILY

Many of the above observations also apply to illness or to loss of another child in the family. The common adult response when serious illness or death of a member of the family is threatened, or when there is a miscarriage or stillbirth, is to attempt to keep such knowledge away from the other children. This is powerfully so where parents, as most do, see their role as being protective and may continue even where children are considerably older, not just in infancy. In reality it is virtually impossible to keep knowledge from siblings as the emotions felt and unwittingly shown by parents inevitably communicate that something is seriously wrong. This may be reinforced by changed behaviour patterns expressed in irritation and anger, or by changed living circumstances within the family as the parents respond to the needs of the sick child.

As previously noted, more distant members of the family may be called in to take over. Thus siblings are separated from the primary source of supportive care and this may generate feelings of rejection. We know separation is a great threat to a child and can sometimes be mirrored in later life and this, in some respect, makes bereavement so difficult to bear throughout later life (Bowlby, 1967).

Siblings often gain knowledge in different ways, such as overhearing phonecalls or part of conversations behind closed doors to which they are inevitably drawn. Information can come from schoolfriends who have heard about the illness in their own homes, often with the instruction 'don't tell anyone', which makes it likely it will be passed on!

This information may be referred to as undigested, or even as indigestible information since knowledge gained cannot be openly acknowledged because of the constraints built into the picture. This means that the knowledge has been worked out with imagination, and without the support and care that would give the child an adequate picture. In some cases the child will build a fantasy picture from the information gained, which may be far removed from reality. The need is to hear the truth spoken with love and care, and with time to understand and help to digest the information. Such openness enables loving care to be shared together within the family and it can be an experience of rich growth for parents and children.

This two-way process between the parents and siblings of the sick child helps to lessen the problems which may occur when pretence is being made. These problems can create distance and cause friction between siblings and parents which may well lead to regressive behaviour problems, which can be interpreted as naughtiness, leading to further isolation. It is common for parents to expect siblings to behave in a way beyond their years at such times when in actual fact they are more likely to be going through a regressive phase of behaviour.

Removal of continuing love, care and support creates insecurity, thus it is necessary to ensure that continuous loving support stays to enable the siblings not only to handle a difficult situation but to continue to develop good relationships with their parents and family.

THE RESPONSE OF PATIENTS TO DEATH ON THEIR WARD

Lasting impressions from messages conveyed

The response of other patients to a death occurring on their ward inevitably hinges on the way in which the death is handled by the staff, the attitudes of the staff and the way in which the practical details are managed.

Example

Procedures such as the way in which the body is removed from the ward can demonstrate, in some circumstances, that the staff are trying to deny that a death has taken place at all. This impression can be given by drawing curtains or lowering lights while the body is removed. One long-term patient was heard to remark 'It's amazing you know that with all that happens on this ward and with all the serious illness, there has not been a single death on the ward', then with a twinkle he added, 'But there have been an awful lot of transfers to other wards!'

The way in which death is handled by staff and in particular whether they communicate the death to fellow patients can have a profound effect on patients. Where there is no direct communication, the patient is left to bear the impact and pain of a death, which may involve a person they have come to know well, and to bear it alone. That there is unwillingness to talk about it puts out a very negative message about death and the way in which the staff view it. Openness and willingness to talk and express sadness at any loss, communicate a sense of their own value to other patients. The value of each patient may well enhance their own self-worth. This approach can communicate a message of hope and reassurance of the kind of care they can expect for themselves.

Where the dying person has been well supported and the individual has been valued, and where the laying out and removal of the body is done with dignity and understanding, a comforting message may well be received by some, if not all, patients from what they have seen and heard.

Response to traumatic events

Some situations are of necessity traumatic, for example, where cardiac arrest has taken place or where a person has died during treatment. There may then be a high level of shock and not a little anxiety and fear concerning what has been seen or heard during the attempt to save the patient's life. Again the knowledge that the highest quality of skill and caring has been given will convey a very positive message. Each patient's own personality together with their present physical, mental, emotional and spiritual state inevitably interacts with what has taken place. Care is needed to try to communicate gently with each patient the facts of the death and to be sensitive to their individual needs. This can be done in such a way that their needs are met rather than denying the facts and thus imposing the agenda of the staff.

Patients frequently form a kind of club to which they belong by reason of shared illness or occupation of a bed in that particular ward. Such a group has its own identity as they begin to take on board the hopes and fears of all the others and become interested in and involved with one another. They come to share hopes and fears, which feed into the nature of their response to a death in their midst. Patients therefore grieve for one another. They may have come to the same clinic and consultant and have seen one another's good and bad moments over the years. They can feel real, deep sense of grief when one of their number dies.

As with some families, there may well be a sense of relief for the other person as their suffering comes to an end. Equally patients can share a deep sense of sadness for the families involved, some of whom they have come to know and like over a period of time. The face of death may seem harsh and difficult and it is part of being human; however, when truth is shared with gentleness and love there is an opportunity for growing in understanding. For many, it may be part of the process of preparation for their own death whether imminent or not.

Strengthening the partnership relationship

The willingness of the staff to share truth honestly and openly with patients is a strong reinforcement of the partnership between patients, families and staff. It can help to create a greater trust so that openness grows with a readiness to explore difficult questions about pain and sadness. To deny truth or to avoid it can make a trusting relationship impossible and will only create more isolation and loneliness.

It is inevitable that the patient's response will be individual even where common factors may be apparent. It is important not only to feed information back but also to listen and respond with sensitivity, giving time so that questions that may be raised by the closeness to death may be worked through as and when other patients feel able and ready. The harsh reality, however, may be that most people of any age cope better with truth than with denial. This does not mean that every patient needs all the truth all of the time and all at once. They should have access and opportunity to explore what it means to them and at a time when they are ready to do so.

> *No man is an island – every man's death diminishes me.*
> John Donne – *Devotions*

QUESTION 1

Each of the following situations may have a different kind of experience for the families and individuals concerned:

(a) Mary is aged 82 and has recently lost her husband. They had been happily married for 50 years and there are two children living abroad.

(b) James and Julia have recently had a second miscarriage and very much want to have a family.

(c) Jimmy who is 5 has cancer. He is likely to live only a few months longer. He has a sister who is 9 years old.

Discuss the nature of the impact of the loss for the individuals concerned and for the other members of their family. Discuss ways in which they can be helped.

QUESTION 2

What particular difficulties may arise for children who have lost a parent, a brother or a sister? How can the effects of the problem be minimised? Discuss this with reference to some of the evidence available.

Key points

- The response to bereavement follows similar patterns to other forms of loss, but the depth and length may be greater.
- The loss of any relationship involves the loss of habits of daily living — a powerfulconsideration in adjustment.
- The death of a parent is the loss of a key relationship.
- The death of a spouse or partner is the loss of a chosen relationship.
- The death of a child reverses the normal order of events.
- The death of a child has a profound effect on siblings.
- Miscarriage and stillbirth have a powerful double impact as the two deeply emotional experiences of birth and death occur together.
- The effects of miscarriage and stillbirth can be as devastating as for a child who has lived, but these facts are often misunderstood.
- The birth of a handicapped child is often associated with strong feelings of guilt
- Adults often underestimate the impact of death on children. Such death can have long-lasting effects and lead to personality problems in later life.
- The response of other patients to a death on the ward can be affected by the way in which staff handle the process.

The patient's response to healing and recovery – new perspectives

*You have freedom to be yourself, your true self here and now
and nothing need stand in your way.*
Richard Bach – *Jonathan Livingston Seagull*

THE HEALING PROCESS – NEW PERSPECTIVES

If you are standing somewhere where the sunlight is falling on a prism, at some moments you will see red flashes of light and at others blue or indigo. Then if you walk around it and the light falls at a different angle you see flashes of yellow or green. Then suddenly the colours vanish for a moment and you see pure white light as they all fuse into one – just for a moment – then it has gone as the individual colours return. So it is when you take a range of different perspectives on a complex subject like spiritual care. It may be necessary to break the picture down into separate components to understand what makes up the whole, but it is as important to stand where you can see the situation as a whole in order to have a greater understanding of all the components.

The last three Chapters have explored in some depth the spiritual response of the patient, client or family to various situations related to sickness and loss. The content of this chapter may appear to repeat some of what has already been discussed and, in one sense, this is so but it is approached from a different perspective. If we are to take a comprehensive look at the whole spectrum of spiritual care, this other perspective will be necessary and helpful at this point.

Some readers will be familiar with the story of Anna – a child with an unusually clear perception of life's realities. Anna says that while most people have many points of view about things, God is different. He has a 'point to view', which is something quite unique (Fynne, 1974).

So here we are looking at response from that more total perspective, in other words from 'a point to view'.

We have looked at the various likely components of response to specific situations and within the experience of one family, several different responses may occur at the same time. For every individual concerned, however, there is a process which takes place over time whatever the circumstances surrounding the person – a process which will involve moving towards death, healing or recovery to a partial or full state of health. Every person passes into and through this process to some extent although the response varies in speed and manner with each individual and situation.

THE RESPONSE TO IMPENDING DEATH

This was discussed in Chapter 8 in the context of the various models of response described by different writers and these are very good examples of the different ways of looking at the same process of approaching impending death. Just as a patient's response may vary in the nature of feelings expressed, so may the perspective of the onlooker or the carer differ in what is observed, recorded or described.

For some, the acceptance of impending death may happen quite quickly with the understanding that the progression of their illness is irreversible. They are prepared to live as fully as possible while preparing themselves and others for their death. For some people, there may be a long period of resistance with fighting or at times apparent recovery before acceptance comes. Acceptance never comes for some people. Whatever the response, it is imperative that each person is allowed to take time to go through the process at their own pace with personal wishes respected without interference and pressure from professionals, family or friends.

THE RESPONSE TO FAILED EXPECTATIONS OF RECOVERY

Most patients have fears of some kind and, for many, there is an unspoken underlying fear of death itself, but at the same time there is often a high level of hope for full recovery. Hope is heightened by an expectation of the medical profession and the treatment offered. Perhaps the first expectation for many is that this is just an interlude in a normal life and once this spell is over they will be able to return to familiar routine again; indeed for many this is what does happen. Here the particular problem can be easily defined, treated, eradicated and cured allowing the patient to return to a little-altered lifestyle.

For others it is clear after a while that a full recovery is not likely. There will be limitations imposed by chronic conditions or by partial removal or loss of a particular function, which has consequences for all aspects of future life, work, social activity and home life. For some there is a need to reach a point of accepting that the implications of the illness are far reaching and will have considerable impact on their lifestyle. Alternatively, it becomes clear that the most likely outcome will be an early death. This may well raise many questions for the patient and family and challenge the hope of recovery to a greater or lesser extent. For the professionals involved, this may bring a need to enter into a different relationship with the patient and family.

The state of mind of the patient in response to the changed circumstances should not set the agenda for the journeying. The state of mind may be affected by the way in which bad news has been communicated and also by the way in which other members of the family or friends respond. As with all aspects of loss, the loss of expectations may trigger many different responses.

There are those who can never acknowledge that recovery will not take place and who will deny the facts from the moment the knowledge is received until they die. They try to live as if the reality experienced is just not true. Some acknowledge the reality and fight with dignity for the best quality of life for as long as possible. There is often a rich experience for them as they develop self-awareness in the fight and new strength in confronting the challenge of the devastation. Others may be able to become acquiescent in accepting the reality of it all and are able to focus on using all their resources on finding a way of living as effectively and fully as is possible. This is different again from those who accept, lose hope and make no attempt to use the time that is left.

Clearly each response makes different demands on the carer in terms of maintaining the dignity and worth of each individual as and where they are. People may move through different responses at different stages of their illness not necessarily consistent with their physical condition, for example the patient may physically be reasonably well but feel utterly dependent. This has implications for the carer who needs to identify where the person stands within himself at a particular time and to come alongside just where the patient is.

Those who find themselves threatened by lack of recovery are in a vulnerable position and at the mercy of those who attempt to offer any form of hope of healing with assurance of recovery. In desperate situations, any avenue is freely entered into and explored, and this should be valued because there is a danger that the presentation of expectations may be too highly positive, raising hopes unrealistically. This can lead to enormous feelings of guilt, frustration, disappointment and resentment against those who have, in all good faith, put forward alternative suggestions or have pressed them to try other methods.

It is clear that no form of therapy or philosophy of healing is universally effective, or everyone would be healed by adopting a particular therapy approach, which clearly does not happen. People respond differently to various forms of healing so it is important that all therapies, treatments and philosophies should be presented with realism and honesty. They all have limitations and can give no guarantee of healing. Many make positive claims for effectiveness that does not always materialise or the claims are more related to the basic comfort of the patient than to recovery. As we shall see in the next paragraph, relationships and trust can play a very important part in this process and this is an aspect of healing which must be recognised and be valued with sensitivity and integrity.

THE RESPONSE TO RECOVERY – SEEKING ALTERNATIVES

Each of us is in truth an idea of the Great Gull, an unlimited idea of freedom, and precision flying is a step towards expressing our real nature ... that's why all this practice ...

Richard Bach – *Jonathan Livingston Seagull.*

Today there is an ever increasing number of complementary therapies and alternative approaches to medical care. Homeopathy and acupuncture have been known and practised for many years while many others have recently joined the list of acceptable therapies, some of which are better than others (Denton and Stevenson, 1992). Popular ones include those like osteopathy, chiropractice, aromatherapy, reflexology and spiritual healing. Therapy also embraces practices including relaxation, visual imagery, meditation and the use of music – many of these already being incorporated into more traditional forms of treatment.

The increase in the use of alternative therapies brings with it an awareness of patients' rights as they become more aware of their own needs and a desire to be treated as a whole person and respected as an individual. There is a growing recognition of the range of choices available and trends in society at large lean towards appreciation of the value of having a choice.

This has been exacerbated for some patients and their families by what can appear at times to be an impersonal approach in traditional medicine. This is highlighted by seeing so many different doctors, having a succession of appointments and by seeing consultants only occasionally with perhaps a few brief moments allocated to them in a busy outpatients department or on a ward round. Clinics and ward rounds often appear formidable with an array of doctors standing around in white coats and talking in a jargon that sounds like another language, all of which makes real access very difficult.

One of the gifts offered by complementary medicine and by its practitioners and therapists is the possibility of entering into a partnership with a single therapist where a significant period of time is allocated for a one-to-one relationship with opportunities for interaction. This, in itself, is a statement of valuation even though it may have been 'bought' for a fee.

Most complementary therapists use touch in one form or another. The use of touch and giving personal attention, together with the opportunity to work together in a partnership, can aid the process of recovery. It may influence the perceived level of pain and may contribute in part to the process of coming to terms with dying through receiving support, care and understanding.

Aromatherapy combines massage (touch) with fragrant oils which often invokes the sense of smell. This has been found increasingly to be valuable in hospices and especially where condition involves unpleasant odours.

The value of personal contact

Clearly an essential ingredient is trusting the therapist and the consequent partnership between patient and therapist. In some areas of medicine, alternative therapies are already incorporated into the range of treatment offered. Others enter into or engage in alternative therapies because of their disappointment with the results achieved by traditional medicine. An important element in this trusting relationship is the inclusion of a positive approach by the patient which is equally valuable for patients who are dying or facing long-term chronic illness as for those whose prospects of recovery are good.

For many, seeking other sources of healing can indicate a strong desire to do something for themselves and can sometimes have an active role in the healing process. Seeking other sources of healing can be an act of desperation driven by fear. Even in these cases, simply the act of giving time, understanding, support and care may help a desperate person to begin the journey towards acceptance of their situation.

The complementary therapies, where well practised, strongly incorporate the value of the spiritual person as well as caring for the body and the patient's condition. For some, they may enable the rediscovery of their own value, dignity and worth. (Rankin–Box, 1988. Byrne, 1992).

Increasingly where tension and stress are concerned, the use of relaxation techniques, meditation of various kinds, hyponosis and visualisation have been shown to have a beneficial effect for a number of patients (Denton, 1992; Pediani, 1992).

As with any treatment or medication, there are those who do not respond well to a particular approach. Part of the art of giving good spiritual care is to respond in the appropriate way for a particular individual and wherever possible to give a choice to the patient.

The patient in control

The need for patients to have a feeling of control over treatment is achieved in conventional medicine in acknowledging the obligation to obtain informed consent before treatment begins. A patient has the right to accept or reject any treatment offered. Again, where a patient wishes to request a particular therapy, effort should be made to provide this unless there are genuine reasons which make it totally inadvisable. There should be very strong reasons for such a request to be denied or heavily discouraged.

It is easy for professional carers to feel threatened by what might appear to be statements that their own care and expertise is inadequate. This is where the second level of partnership between the various disciplines is needed as well as a generosity of spirit to accept and allow a particular therapy or approach to be used. The therapy may be beneficial or important to the patient simply because the patient values it. The power of the mind should never be underestimated.

Control is two way: the patient should have control so that if the carer offers a particular therapy which is not acceptable he or she has the right to refuse. Equally, there is the right to ask for other therapies or for another person to provide support through their presence, counselling or prayer. These wishes should be complied with even if this is outside the accepted practices of a practitioner or carer's parameters of experience and understanding, or contrary to the carer's belief and practice.

The carer has no need to participate and indeed has the right of conscience not to participate in any practice they find objectionable, but to deny that practice to another, unless it can be shown to be detrimental to the patient or others or to be against the law, would be a denial of rights and contrary to the Patients' Charter.

Finally, one reason for the patient's request for a certain alternative therapy may well be that it is possible for members of the family or trusted friends to be involved with their administration. This is particularly so with treatments involving massage or aromatherapy, or where experiences can be shared as in practices such as meditation or visualisation.

RESPONSE TO RECOVERY

It is an appropriate reminder that happily for the majority of patients recovery is complete or relatively so, and it can be expected that they will return to their former style of living and leave behind the interlude of sickness as soon as possible. There are occasions, however, where individuals respond by adopting a completely new lifestyle. They may want a change to a more relaxed way of life, or choose a more satisfying or less stressful occupation. They may well decide they are grateful for renewed strength and health, that they have found a new sense of purpose and decide to seek a fuller and more varied way of living. They may decide to travel more or to spend more time with the family. All these changes may make demands on their friends or family and have far-reaching implications with adjustments to follow.

This is a very valid point at which to leave our exploration of the patient's response and to bring together the carer's resources and the patient's needs in responding to illness·as in the next section we look at the kind of provision made to offer a service in spiritual care.

EXERCISE 22

Take a look again at your answers to the Questions sections at the end of Chapter 8. Discuss some of your conclusions in your group, after reading this Chapter. Look at any personal experiences members wish to share and at the use of alternative therapies.
Look again at the advantages and disadvantages in the light of the current evidence available and after looking at some of the references given. Revise these from time to time as further knowledge and experience becomes available.

EXERCISE 23

This is a personal recapitulation for you at the end of Section III. Summarise any changes in your own perspective on ways in which patients respond to recovery. How has this broadened your awareness of and sensitivity to spiritual need?

Key points

- To look at some issues from a different perspective is valuable.
- Patients respond in different ways to impending death or failed expectations.
- Response to illness and recovery may involve seeking alternative therapies.
- It is important that the patient's wishes are recognised and valued.
- These therapies give the family a chance to be involved with care and can be a learning experience for them also.
- Carers need to beware of imposing their own beliefs on patients.
- Some patients who recover completely return to normal life. Others find renewed purpose for living and may seek a change of lifestyle.

Section IV

Provision for meeting special needs in particular situations

What are our lives but harbours
we are continually setting out
from, airports at which we touch
down and remain in too briefly –
And always in one
another we seek the proof
of experiences it would be worth dying for.
RS Thomas – *Somewhere*

In the last two Sections, we have explored in some depth the resources, needs and responses of two participants (that is the patient or client and the carer) in the partnership which is so central to the provision of spiritual care. For that relationship to be really effective, it needs to offer a comfortable and supportive framework in an environment conducive to good communication and one in which the partnership can grow and develop.

This whole Section focuses on that environment, concentrating on special provisions within organisations and the community to facilitate the meeting of particular needs in different situations. While the overall provision is important, the previous Chapter clearly showed the range of variations in needs and responses in different departments such as obstetrics, intensive care, or geriatrics so the kind of provision needed will vary accordingly.

We also explore wider issues influencing the provision of spiritual care such as the need to respect and make provision for different religious beliefs and practices or cultural customs. This includes consideration of general cultural influences and attitudes towards current social and health related problems such as drug addiction or AIDS. The Section concludes by looking at some ethical issues facing carers and patients where personal values and beliefs may raise areas of conflict which need openness and sensitivity to resolve.

We must remember that while we explore these wider issues we still need to have as our primary focus the nurturing and development of that sensitive caring relationship, which is the core of spiritual care.

EXERCISE 24

As you read through this Section, make a note of any particular provisions for spiritual care you have in your own workplace or specialist units and keep this until the Questions section at the end of each Chapter. It will be useful to compare these with notes from colleagues in different professions or centres.

CHAPTER 12

Provision for meeting particular spiritual needs – unexpected situations and general principles

Those who listen day after day – in exposing themselves to another's pain are part of the healing process.

Sheila Cassidy – *Good Friday People*

Some aspects of spiritual care are common to all situations and can be seen to be a normal part of the provision of spiritual care by healthcare professionals. These aspects have a place in the education and training courses of healthcare workers. There is a need to develop these aspects of the work further to enhance the appropriate skills. This is especially important when meeting situations which are particularly demanding.

Some areas of work such as intensive care or accident and emergency units have a strong element of shock involved in the response of patients and relatives. These need special skill and provision to allow relatives to receive bad news and begin the process of coming to terms with the information and its consequences. Miscarriage, stillbirth or the death of a child are examples of situations which, by their nature, are shattering experiences causing deep shock. Although shock is part of the response in any situation involving death or the communication of bad news, sudden death often creates a particularly powerful shock response because of its unexpectedness.

It is often forgotten that many sick people are cared for at home and indeed a significant number die at home.

GENERAL PROVISIONS

Apart from the provision of spiritual care by the nursing and medical staff, there are other relevant services available such as the care from a chaplaincy department, which can help with a wide range of needs. Other forms of care come through occupational therapy or alternative medicine practices. There are support groups both in the hospital and the community which are available for a range of special needs and bring immense relief to carers and patients, putting them in touch with others suffering in similar situations. These are discussed in detail in a later Chapter, but it is particularly important here to note their value in assisting patients and families to come to terms with and to cope with the experience of illness, disability or loss.

To make our exploration easier to follow, this Chapter groups together those areas where provision needs to take account of sudden death, injury and shock. The following Chapter looks at those needing longer term care, often in the community, and considers approaches to providing a response to some social problems related to incapacity and ill health.

BEREAVEMENT

Spiritual care of the bereaved is an important and sensitive area which has often been neglected. While different wards and departments need to take account of their own particular circumstances, it is also important to have a recognised procedure in the organisation as a whole. Evidence suggests that such provision varies widely and a recent study by Jackson shows there is a generally low level of after care for bereaved families and friends (Jackson, 1992). The study covered senior sisters/charge nurses in intensive care units in the UK and of 83 respondents, 49 had no follow-up service at all. Only 10 provided a structured service of any kind with access to a bereavement specialist (*see also* the King's Fund Study, 1990).

It is increasingly becoming recognised that special skills are involved and that relatives need privacy and quietness in which to express their feelings away from the scene of the recent traumatic events. Ward staff also need to be relieved of the administrative aspects surrounding the death, as these are more appropriately dealt with by others who have special knowledge and access to the right people and resources. There is growing awareness that some kind of Bereavement Centre is the best way to provide for these needs. Different kinds of provision are being set up locally according to the resources and needs available but, as yet, this concept is much in its infancy.

An example of a Bereavement Centre service

After the Kegworth air disaster, the experience gained in making special provision for bereaved families and relatives at the Queen's Medical Centre was found to be valuable in establishing a Bereavement Centre service, adjacent to the chaplaincy department and managed by the senior chaplain. Here the bereaved relatives are referred from the wards and brought to a comfortably furnished centre where they can find peace and privacy. The necessary details are dealt with efficiently and sympathetically by skilled administrative staff who have immediate access to local information and organisational resources. If requested, arrangements can be made for the relatives to speak with the doctor who has been involved with the patient or to talk with a chaplain or anyone else they ask to see. There are also local volunteers who have special skills in listening and who are available to provide refreshments or to escort bewildered relatives wherever they need to go in the building.

❧

Centre staff are committed to providing caring support to relatives in this relaxed and comfortable setting, and are sensitive to the needs of all faiths and cultures. People who have been bereaved often phone or drop in to the centre later on for further care and help and, where appropriate, regular support and counselling are provided. In addition to routine administrative services, staff are able to advise on more complicated situations such as procedures for donating organs to medical science or for taking bodies out of the country. They maintain links with and current information on self-help groups and many outside agencies such as Cruse, Sands, or AIDS Bereavement Support.

The centre also has a role to provide an educative and supportive service for staff. Routine placements are arranged for students, staff nurses and many other professionals on specialist courses within the hospital and local community. Courses can be arranged to prepare them to cope with the difficult bereavement situations and the personal trauma which they themselves constantly face. Volunteers also need special training for dealing with bereaved people and thus there is a 'ripple effect' of spreading new attitudes and understanding about a subject which is so often difficult to talk about. The centre is also able to refer those who request or need further counselling and support to local professionals.

There are strong similarities between responses to bereavement in all areas and an overall policy is ideal. Nevertheless, there are particular aspects of response from patients and relatives that are highlighted by the nature of the situation. In the previous Chapter some common aspects of response were discussed, describing the profound element of shock and disbelief accompanying sudden death, which is particularly intense owing to its unexpected nature.

This is especially so with the death of children or younger people where there is an expectation of many years of life ahead and where other young family members may be involved in a particularly intense way. While feelings are intense in all bereavements, there is clearly a need to make special provision for the more traumatic situations. Such unexpected deaths are most likely to occur in obstetrics, paediatrics, accident and emergency, or in intensive care units, so we will focus on each of these areas in turn.

THE OBSTETRIC DEPARTMENT

Here we have an example of an area where special needs are very obvious and there is a general public expectation of specific support. The provision needs to be seen in the context of the paragraphs in the previous Chapter describing the very specific response to this kind of bereavement. It is a situation where there have been high hopes of a new life and so shock is very intense and, in particular, there is the loss of the anticipated nurturing role and therefore there is a very painful response. This demands an extremely sensitive policy with facilities for holding the baby and for clear recognition of the significance of the birth at whatever stage of pregnancy the loss has occurred (Hopper, 1991; Thomas, 1992).

Even in early miscarriage where there is no recoverable foetus, it is still important for many parents to be able to mark the significance of what has taken place, perhaps by arranging for the child to have a name and a funeral with a coffin. For others it is sufficient to have the opportunity to participate in a service of some kind where they can express their pain, loss and sadness, and express in a tangible way the love that is already there and which has been so powerfully and abruptly cut off. There can be immense value derived from participation in an occasion which gives lasting significance to the event. Others will appreciate the opportunity to have an entry in a book of remembrance – something which offers a visual focus or something tangible to see and touch from time to time. To be able to write a personal note or message in that place can help to express grief and pain in a positive way. In the later stages of miscarriage or stillbirth, it is of course possible to have a funeral in the traditional way. Attention is increasingly being focused on memorabilia in the form of footprints, handprints, photos and entries in books of remembrance and so on marking the event or service (Stewart *et al.*, 1992)

This is something which may sometimes create a strong anti-reaction for some of the family who take the line 'forget it all – put it all behind you and have another quickly'. Evidence shows that attempts to repress painful experiences in this way can create considerable suffering over a long period of time. There is a helpful significance sometimes in dressing the baby in ordinary clothes that have been lovingly prepared and in holding the baby for a photo, then placing with a cuddly toy in the coffin. All these things are important in the process of grieving as they give the baby a personality and a name by which he or she can be remembered and mourned. Both Hopper (1991) and Thomas (1991) have written detailed accounts of the kind of specialist services they have developed in this area.

While it is important to make as many options available as possible, it is essential that the staff involved see them as choices for the parents and do not impose them. Some want everything to be simple and some want more time alone with their baby.

Example
Perhaps this example will act as a salutary lesson. The day after the death of their baby, the parents returned to see the baby in the mortuary. They were clearly very tense and anxious. I explained as we went what we would find and offered them the choices of having me with them for all or part of the time, and of when the naming and blessing of the baby would happen. They looked somewhat surprised and said 'Do you mean that?' After that the parents were very open with many tears. The mother then said 'We feel we now have our baby back. Yesterday we felt just like bit players in the staff's drama!'

PAEDIATRICS DEPARTMENT

The devastation accompanying the death of a child has already been discussed in Chapter 10. The severance of the parental role has a powerful impact as it embodies memories of a life already lived together and an abrupt loss of future hopes. Again an area which needs a special sensitivity on the part of the staff, is the creation of a caring environment where parents can remain for a while and take their time to assimilate what has happened. This is particularly so where a baby or child is taken off a life support machine when it is important to ensure the last moments of the short life are handled with dignity and sensitivity. At the same time, care must be taken to avoid over-managing the situation, rushing it, turning it into a drama or a weepy situation, or play-acting (Hopper, 1991; Thomas, 1991).

The loss of a child is a harsh reality and attempts to make it anything other than that are dangerous as they tend to take away any of the reality of the situation. There is a need for clear demonstration and recognition that the dead child is a part of the family – the child of parents, and the brother or sister of siblings. As far as possible, privacy is necessary, with or without the presence of staff, so that the family can be themselves and say and do what needs to be said and done.

Again, memorabilia such as photographs, locks of hair or items belonging to the child are of importance. Some units have moved a long way towards involving parents in all aspects of care in illness and in death. For example, they can share in the dispensation of drugs where the drugs come from the parents' hands instead of the staff but they need staff support and help. Parents can be involved with the laying out of the child with considerable benefit to themselves and staff – it is the last act of care they can offer their child apart from the funeral itself. All this allows them to express significance rather divesting it of value and importance (Burgess, 1992).

Reference to local support groups is often helpful and many organisations such as Compassionate Friends, or Cruse are available to give local support.

ACCIDENT AND EMERGENCY

> *Go placidly amid the noise and haste and remember what peace*
> *there may be in silence. As far as possible without surrender be*
> *on good terms with all persons. Speak your truth quietly*
> *and clearly and listen to others*
>
> Found in St Paul's Church, Baltimore – *Desiderata*

Large accident and emergency departments tend to see an enormous number of traumatic events, including sudden deaths and major injuries. These entail dramatic moments in an area vibrant with activity. For families or friends involved, this situation has come as an intense shock, with the realisation that the patient was involved in an accident or sudden illness and has arrived in an area where intense treatment is given with urgency. This all fuels the rage and disbelief and the levels of shock are very high, with a whole range of responses from anger and hysteria to withdrawal. Directness with sensitivity in breaking news is important – as in shock little can be taken in so information needs to be simple (that is with no jargon) and pithy.

Surroundings may not be ideal for creating a reassuring atmosphere. It is the attitudes of staff, however, which are most important in helping families to encounter the harsh realities of life and death. Despite the distractions going on around and the unusual activity, it is possible to create a quiet atmosphere and lend dignity and privacy to the moment. It is always important to be aware that the vast majority of people have no experience of the type of equipment used or of treatment given in this strange environment. They therefore need preparation before going into a cubicle and support is vital.

It is important to allow opportunity for physical contact, for holding or kissing after a sudden death, and for farewells to be taken. Where staff feel able, it helps for them to hold the shattered relative if appropriate. It can help to write down what has happened as shocked relatives often fail to grasp the significance of events which have occurred, or to arrange a chance for them to return at a later time to talk over what has happened with the person involved in the event to allow for questions and response (Burgess, 1992). Frequently, people who have been spoken to when shocked have not been able to engage with what has been said and later feel resentful and that they have not been told anything.

INTENSIVE CARE AND CORONARY CARE

This is another area where there may be an element of unexpectedness contributing to deep shock. This can happen when patients are admitted directly from accident and emergency, or after surgery or sudden collapse on a ward creating a life-threatening situation, or where relatives are suddenly presented with a gloomy prognosis. In each case the threat of death is part of the picture. Again it is important to recognise the threatening situation created for a relative by being surrounded by high technology in the form of unfamiliar machinery, which takes over the normal functions of life and monitoring conditions. All of this can have a profound effect on those who are unfamiliar with such procedures. Whether the patient recovers fully, partially or returns to the ward, there may be indications of changed personality so staff are struggling with families who are themselves struggling to come to terms with repeated shocks and changes in condition.

Staff need to take especial care over the way in which information is shared as people often fail to take in what is said and it may need reinforcing several times.

As relatives' own belief patterns may be threatened, there is a need for support and much empathy during explanation. It is important to constantly remain firm to the known diagnosis or outcome, even when under pressure to put more into the picture than the facts warrant or to offer false hopes. It is common for families to do the rounds of staff attempting to extract a more hopeful picture.

With all the bustle and activity in an atmosphere created by high technology and urgency, a place of quiet is an essential provision, where families can get away from the visual impact of high technology and the constant threat of death and receive care themselves. This is a place where they can reflect and come to terms with what is happening and face the impact of possible death. There needs to be an atmosphere of trust with the staff so they can feel free to ask questions and come back for further information as they are ready to accept it, or to hear the truth repeated again, or have the diagnosis clarified or confirmed (Burgess, 1992).

Clearly in this area of high activity there is also a need for recognition of the needs of staff to attend to their own spiritual care, and their welfare should be safeguarded in the way in which this is managed. Their pressures need to be recognised, accepted and adequate support should be available (see Chapters 17 and 18).

Where there is likely to be a lengthy stay in the intensive care unit, provision of a different kind may be necessary as the pressures do not only relate to bereavement.

SPIRITUAL CARE IN MAJOR DISASTERS

There are two major aspects of provision to consider here: provision of care at the site of disaster; and also in the reception areas where care is given at the hospital.

Coping with the unexpected

Major disasters, by their very nature, have an element of chaos in the immediate situation. Whatever happens and wherever the event occurs, no one is ready waiting for it and there is always an element of surprise. No matter how many plans are made or dummy runs held (and these are important), each time the situation is unique and the reality is different and unexpected.

This element of the unexpected in itself creates a measure of shock and surprise for people at the site of the disaster, for the emergency services, for those in the reception areas at the hospital, and for the neighbourhood and nation concerned. There is much activity involved in immediate response at the site of the accident which has to be spontaneous. This may involve onlookers who are unprepared as well as the emergency services who have little warning of the size or nature of involvement, and who have to make quick decisions positively prioritising about the order of rescue.

For those who are responding to the immediate needs, whatever their capacity or responsibility, they are working at the limits of their physical and mental resources with a massive amount of adrenaline flowing. They are having to make quick decisions in conditions far from ideal, and snap judgements on life-and-death issues, sometimes with choices between two equally difficult options. This is true for both site activities and hospital care in the accident and emergency and the immediate receiving areas.

Provision for staff care

Added pressures arise for the teams at work when the media come, and later with visits from other dignitaries, which result in the patients, staff and relatives being constantly under intense scrutiny. The urgency of the situation and increased flow of adrenaline enables staff to keep going to extraordinary lengths and this needs to be watched with care by each individual and by those with management responsibility. It is an important aspect of spiritual care for the carers to ensure staff do not work continuously without proper refreshment, rest and immediate debriefing care and support (McKinlay, 1991; Paton, 1990).

There is a need for informal debriefing on the spot, more formal debriefing sessions for all staff concerned and arrangements for follow-up support and counselling where necessary for a further period of time in order to minimise the effects of post-traumatic stress syndrome. (This is explored more fully in Chapter 18.)

Part of the pressure comes from being faced with very severe injuries, not just singly but in a multiple form, which adds to the powerful impact on the responding teams. While they are professionals trained to handle such injuries, they are still individuals with human responses and feelings which must be respected and they need adequate support.

Provision for general debriefing

Post-traumatic stress syndrome can affect not only staff, but immediate families of victims and even members of extended families, and also onlookers who were perhaps the first to arrive on the scene and are often forgotten (Woodruffe, 1989; Mitchell, 1983). Victims who have been caught up in disaster in any way and looked death closely in the face or who, looking around them, have seen death in its ugliness and reality, need to be enabled to talk through their feelings as soon as possible and to receive a response to those feelings. They need to be able to go over recent events again and again with all the horror or trivialities. They also need to look at the possible consequences for themselves and their families, all of whom may be in severe shock and in danger of having their pain 'gobbled up' by the media and publicised (Gibson, 1991).

Space and privacy

Provision is thus needed for quiet space and privacy where people can talk freely with dignity and with complete confidentiality. They need skilled help to explore and work through the situation, however painful, and to move on to reconstruction for the future. It is of utmost importance for all involved to have this facility. Indeed, the spiritual experience of realising and acknowledging the horror of raw suffering and exploring it in the context of love and a caring relationship can build up a picture of sharp contrasts, which, in itself, can be a creative experience. When expressed, contrasting and extreme feelings often come very close together: fear and despair live next to hope and expectations; love and hate are juxtaposed closely together; and expressions of anger can be followed by a quiet acceptance and sense of peace. Such an exploration can create very close bonds between the carer or rescuer and the victim and family involved.

Self development and preparation for support

Only too often there is a meticulous and well-publicised preparation for the organisational and administrative aspects of management of major incidents which, important as it is, overlooks some of the human factors involved. There is a need for preliminary staff development and training for all likely to be involved at whatever level; however, this is a less spectacular kind of preparation and its significance is often missed. There also needs to be structured care built into the system for those whose

role is the care of anyone involved, especially those who are not directly involved with physical care or the 'doers' (Owen et al., 1989).

This includes those whose task is the emotional, social, religious or spiritual care, which in a sense can wrap itself around the whole situation and bring an essential sense of peace to much of the care. Many people can be involved with this as they are all in some way affected – the families of staff, local volunteers, groups and churches may well have a role to play.

There may be a need for more than one place of safety for staff in their needs and for friends and relatives, not forgetting that the victims also have needs for a place to unload in privacy. The place of safety is met initially with the attitudes of the rescuers and then those from people in the reception areas where casualties or relatives first arrive in the hospital. It is also experienced in the 'presence' of the carers through their expertise and ability to deal with immediate physical needs. This is evident through their approach as they recognise and accept spiritual needs and offer appropriate spiritual care which accepts the person, gives value and dignity to those in need and demonstrates a willingness to be exposed to the raw experience of devastating injury, shock and suffering.

As patients are moved on through the system, these facilities need to be available with continuity throughout the care process. There is need for places where everyone concerned can find a space for exploration, so that they can move forward into understanding and acceptance. Above all it is people who provide a place of safety!

Spiritual care provision for relatives

The need for special provisions for relatives who may have to be around for some time should not be overlooked. Experience gained in major disaster situations such as those after the Kegworth air crash or the Hillsborough disaster highlighted these needs as families often have to travel from some distance away. Their immediate need is for a place where they can go and get first-hand information about the victim, and the system needs to have clear and efficient organisation here (Gibson, 1991).

Example
The way this is done will vary according to local facilities but in Queen's Medical Centre at Nottingham a team of chaplains, social workers, nurses and selected volunteers was set up for this purpose. The team was able to facilitate arrangements to ensure relatives had whatever information was available speedily, accurately and directly from the units concerned. The carers also provided for their physical needs such as refreshment and rest, once they were secure in the knowledge that they would be able to be taken directly to the victim as soon as was practicable. In this way a considerable load was taken away from the staff who were fully occupied in coping with a vast influx of seriously ill patients. Accurate information given in a caring accepting environment does much to alleviate the inevitable shock which families experience.

Provision for after care

The need for a structured approach to spiritual care does not cease once the immediate crisis is over. There is often a need to make arrangements for further support during a period of adjustment as patients and families return home. This is where good liaison with a support service and groups in the community is essential to ensure the continuity of care throughout the recovery period. It may well be possible to hand over to local groups, friends or professionals to continue the care, or the family unit may be able to provide its own care and there are yet others who will need skilled professional help for months or years to come (Stoter, 1989).

QUESTION 1
Describe in detail the provisions for spiritual care of the bereaved relatives in:
(a) Your own organisation as a whole.
(b) Your own present sphere of work.
Now suggest ways in which you think they can be improved giving your reasons. (Use any notes you have made while reading this Chapter)

QUESTION 2
Outline the special provisions required for spiritual care of patients and families in two of the following units:
(a) Obstetrics
(b) Paediatrics
(c) Accident and emergency
(d) Intensive care unit
Identify the special needs in each section.

QUESTION 3
A major disaster can have far reaching effects not only for victims but also for many others involved peripherally. Discuss some of the immediate and long-term effects on anyone associated and outline the important provision for spiritual care.

Key points

- As there are many responses to pain and suffering, so there must be a variety of appropriate provisions for spiritual care.
- A bereavement centre is an efficient way of providing a sensitive service and using resources properly.
- Special provisions are essential for bereaved parents to come to terms with miscarriage and stillbirth, or the death of a child, with special funeral provisions and use of memorabilia.
- Major disasters need special preparations and an inbuilt system for training staff and for debriefing purposes.
- Proper preparations can do much to lessen the effects of post traumatic stress syndrome.

13

Provision for spiritual needs – long-term situations

To cure sometimes
To relieve often
To comfort always.

Strauss – in Franklin, *Medical Quotations*

LONG-STAY PATIENTS, COMMUNITY AND SOCIAL CARE

Bereavement is a devastating experience whenever and in whatever situation it occurs. There can be situations, however, in which there is a long and perhaps weary period of anticipation, which for some relatives is a time which may allow some preparation for the death and time to share with the person who is terminally ill.

There are also other aspects of long-term illness where death is not necessarily imminent, but there may be a long period of incapacity stretching ahead. These situations need sensitive approaches to spiritual care requiring separate provisions to be built into the care. Such provisions may be necessary to improve the patient's quality of life. Much of this time may well be spent at home where community staff have a vital role both directly with the patients and also with helping family and friends to play their part and so to avoid the spiritual isolation that can occur when family and friends deny the opportunity to explore feelings.

The following paragraphs will be presented with that assumption, that special ongoing provision may be needed to provide continuity as the patient moves away from the hospital setting.

SPIRITUAL HEALTH FOR LONG-STAY PATIENTS

There is always an element of shock attached to bereavement, even when the death has been anticipated for some while. The spiritual care of those who are ill for a long period of time is important and demanding. It is important to try to ensure the quality of life remaining for the patient and family. The spiritual care offered may involve preparation for possible changes in lifestyle or adaptation to the knowledge of gradual physical deterioration or impending death.

In these situations different aspects of ongoing care need recognition, for example, support groups either in the hospital or continuing into the community and home afterwards. There are many such groups organised in some cases through the relevant hospital or unit. In other cases such as oncology, multiple sclerosis or loss of sight, there are often local branches of specialist charities offering voluntary and/or expert help through individuals or support groups. These groups may bring the individual or family concerned into touch with others who are coping with similar problems and so are a means of providing strength, encouragement, practical help and guidance.

SPIRITUAL CARE FOR THE ELDERLY

Beatitudes for the elderly

Blessed are they who understand
My faltering steps and shaking hand
Blessed, they who know my ears today
Must strain to catch the things they say.
Blessed are they with a cheery smile
Who stop to chat for a little while.
Blessed are they who never say
'You've told that story twice today'.
Blessed are they who make it known
That I'm loved, respected and not alone.

Barbara Beuler Wegner (source unknown)

Although illness, incapacity and impending death may appear to be a natural part of old age, the impact of ageing may be alleviated considerably by increased medical care and healthcare, and consequently expectations of a longer active life are high. Many conditions which would previously have been terminal can now be treated. In these situations there is a continuous need for a high quality of spiritual care to be available over what may be a considerable period of time. Many elderly folk may have had experience of being separated from their partner for a while, perhaps through previous illness or war, while some are facing this prospect for the first time.

This may mean facing loneliness when they had come to expect and rely on sharing life together. Others may be faced with seeing a relative who, as in Alzheimer's disease, was once a capable and caring intelligent person and is now no longer able to communicate and presents a totally changed personality. Similar problems arise after severe strokes bringing intense pain to those who care – especially to partners, family and friends.

The spiritual care of the family needs special thought – often they need to be listened to again and again even when the same stories are being repeated telling how important the sick person has been to the partner, family and the community. For patients who can communicate, there may be a need to talk constantly and repeatedly about their past and this is often where a friendly visitor or a volunteer helper can offer a useful back-up to the ward team or, if at home, to the family. This is simply someone to listen to the expression of pain and loneliness or perhaps to look at old photographs as they recall past memories. The process of recall of important memories may often be an attempt to prove to others and to the family and to themselves that their life has been valuable. Sometimes the impending death may cause recall of a memory, or memories, which may have been buried and repressed for many years.

Example
For example, a man who had served in the RAF as a wartime bomb aimer became very troubled by his memories as he faced his own death. He shared the memories of many raids over enemy cities and said, 'I had to do it – I knew there were women and children down there – we had to steel ourselves to do it to build up a kind of hatred inside. When I pressed the button I used to scream "Burn you – burn!" He needed to explore this at length together with the rest of his life. He did find peace and the forgiveness he felt he needed and died very peacefully.

It is a fallacy to believe that old people cope better with illness, death and ageing, and bereavement. The phrase, 'He or she has had a good innings' is meaningless and often offensive for many people as however many years companionship has been shared, there is always the hope that it will continue for some further years. For younger members of a family, facing the death of parents may bring their own awareness of mortality closer.

For elderly patients needing longer-term care, it is important to make provision for them to retain contact with the outside or real world for as long as possible. This can be accomplished through being taken out, through visiting the family at intervals or through arranging flexible visiting arrangements for family and friends. Often babies and children can provide that essential touch of normality so much needed to prevent them from losing touch with the real world.

It is important to keep all avenues open. For people who are deaf or blind, in particular, the use of other senses can be encouraged for communication. One example of this is the increasing use of music therapy or, where appropriate, introducing friendly animals for patients to touch. Many older people respond readily to this kind of communication. It is essential to keep all channels open in order to retain the patient's capacity to relate to carers and respond to life and the normal world. This facility can also be helped by retaining some of their loved personal possessions around them where possible. Other aids available include taped books for those who are blind or partially sighted, or who can no longer hold a book to read. It often takes time and imagination to find out what individual patients might use, but it pays dividends in terms of keeping their facility to relate. It is also important not to assume that we know what patients enjoy. Several elderly patients have said, 'I hate Bingo, but they (the staff) think you are being awkward if you do not join in.'.

EXERCISE 25

Long-stay patients pose a challenge to carers for the provision of spiritual care. Explore any innovative schemes or ideas you know of and also the reasons for meeting the needs of this often neglected group.

TERMINAL CARE

Terminal care may be provided within a general or specialist unit. The patient may be transferred to hospice care or be nursed at home with specialist help from the home care team. There is a significant relationship between spirituality and wellbeing during terminal illness, which makes an important contribution to the patient's quality of life (Reed, 1987). One important issue to consider is that whatever the nature of the illness, the patient will have reached a stage on the spiritual journey at his own pace and in relation to his individual experience. People journey in different ways and this needs to be recognised and accepted by all carers. The provision of spiritual care needs to be matched to the agenda and needs of the patient and not to the agenda prescribed by the carer.

An area needing a fine balancing act is where what the patient needs and wants has to be brought into some kind of coherence with the family needs. The family might be experiencing a strong compulsion to impose their own agenda on the patient, and feel fear, guilt or frustration when this is not being accepted. Families may need expert help to communicate support for the patient, to understand the real need and to cope with their own feelings of rejection if these offers of help are not wanted. There is no worse legacy than failure to communicate, which can block a relationship. This is often evident when the patient is denied access to information which the family has and when issues which need to be shared and discussed together are avoided deliberately.

Whatever happens it is important to avoid over-cosseting patients and making decisions for them. It is essential to allow time for them to reach their own decisions and not to be rushed into premature action. Sometimes families are too anxious to take over responsibilities when the sick person might well be able to continue with some areas of activity which will bring a sense of being worthwhile and bring value to their life for as long as possible.

Example

Jane, once a very active person, had become blind and partially paralysed for many years after a viral infection and her incapacity left her depressed and frustrated. One of the staff discovered she had some movement in her little finger and was able to get her fixed up with a specially adapted typewriter. (There were no computers in her day.) She was then able to write several letters daily, which gave her great satisfaction as this became her one means of communication with the outside world and allowed her a degree of autonomy and independence which she cherished. She was able to write letters for fellow patients and run her own correspondence club, which gave her a new purpose in life and became a joy to many others as well until she died.

SPIRITUAL CARE IN THE COMMUNITY

The need for continuity in the provision of spiritual care for those nursed at home is just as important to consider. Community care is often ongoing for a longer period of time and within the context of a relationship which offers opportunities for assessment of spiritual need and long-term planning for care (Burkhardt and Nasai-Jacoban, 1985).

Patients and families may again need access to some expert assistance to maintain relationships and a good quality of life. A special difficulty here for patients and carers is isolation where they often feel neglected or inadequately supported for the role they have to play. This is at a time when relationships are vital and the level of communication can easily be adversely affected. The sheer weight of extra work in terms of shopping, washing or attention to care may limit the time available for listening or just a chat in passing as the carers become exhausted. The value of support groups with special interests or voluntary visitors, as noted earlier, is very apparent.

Inevitably, the professional carers involved tend to focus on the medical and nursing care, but it is important and possible to build time for listening and responding to the needs of the patient and family into the care process. Frequently, the anxiety to protect the patient may limit the avenues of communication and cause tensions leading to guilt and irritation (Owen, 1989). Attention given in this way often saves time and anxiety. The knowledge that time will be given freely when needed can help to make a patient less demanding.

The need for respite is important here. This need not only mean taking the patient into hospital or hospice care, but includes other forms of relief for relatives, such as a few hours off to sleep, to go out to tea with friends or to the park for a walk. This is an area which will require much more provision as the effects of demographic changes are felt with an ageing population.

There is ample opportunity here for local groups, charities and churches to be involved. Professionals can take a greater initiative in encouraging such liaisons, as the policy to increase community care becomes more widely established.

Volunteers need some preparation and training from professional experts, but with increasing numbers of people retiring early, many are capable and would welcome an opportunity to give the kind of befriending which may be needed. They need guidance, support and some preparation, however, if they are not to become overwhelmed by the impact of suffering. Some church workers may need guidance in this aspect of visiting to cope with their own approach to listening and to avoid proselytising. Professional staff also need help if they feel threatened by a loss of professional role. There may, in addition, be benefit to local organisations and groups in raising their own levels of skill and drawing individuals closer together, thus enhancing community life. The provision of good spiritual care enables providers, as well as the receivers, to benefit from the interdependence created by relationships.

EXERCISE 26
Discuss within your group some examples of the need for spiritual care in the community.
• Identify the various groups needing care.

- Examples of ways in which there is good provision locally and nationally.
- Identify the issues which tend to be overlooked because they are time consuming and difficult to deal with.

PROVISION FOR SPIRITUAL CARE FOR HIV AND AIDS PATIENTS

There are many different issues facing those who are diagnosed as HIV-positive and AIDS. These issues need recognition whether the kind of care needed is as an inpatient in hospital or in a hospice, or ongoing community care. In many cases there is a strong desire for secrecy and confidentiality and this is a factor which must be respected. There is now a growing number of support groups offering specialist help to all the victims. Throughout the country, there are strong links between the groups and hospitals involved with care.

Issues to be faced vary with the patient's condition, family support and local acceptance. A patient who has been diagnosed as HIV positive may be living with uncertainty for many years and need to adjust to a situation of coming to terms with living with this knowledge. By contrast, someone who is in an advanced stage of AIDS is needing help to come to terms with the possibility of increasing illness and incapacity, with limited hope of treatment available. So some are learning to live with their problem, while others face dying with it.

In addition, many will have to face some aspects of stigma or prejudice from society, friends or family. The family themselves may well need help to adjust to the shock on receiving the information. Therefore, one of the most important needs is to provide help in overcoming the fears and prejudices surrounding these conditions for the caring professions and for the community at large to bring normality into the care. The condition affects an increasingly wide spectrum of society. Some may have had relationships which have been severed abruptly or changed on account of the disease because of prejudice or fear. One of the most important needs is to bring a sense of normality to the situation while recognising the enormity of the patient's shock and suffering, exacerbated by having a disease which as yet has no apparent cure.

There is a need to provide for the full range of response already described relating to shock and uncertainty, and to allow for time and space to sit with the patient. It is important to listen, share, touch and hold and to understand without being judgmental. For some, there is a particular need (not unique to this situation, of course) to assist reconciliation within an alienated family. This does not mean that alienation always follows – some have particularly supportive families and close relationships may be enhanced through the sharing of suffering.

Part of the process of valuing is the ability to offer choices to the sufferer and to the family, building a partnership which is so important in this kind of care.

Another important area of provision needed, is to help society at large to come to terms with fears and some wilder misconceptions about the disease and its transmission. This is often best done through the input of local groups who have accurate information to communicate. One particularly good example of media education has been through the programme of *Eastenders* over recent years. The sensitive handling of the issues and confrontation of fears and prejudices within a popular television programme has enabled many viewers to assimilate knowledge and to change attitudes.

Much of the best provision is given by specialist treatment centres, increasingly from local units offering individual counselling support to patients and families. There are also support groups where they can feel accepted and at ease with others in similar situations and with those who have developed awareness and sensitivity to the problems experienced. Details of some national organisations and charitable groups are to be found at the end of this book and reference to these can provide local information.

One aspect which should not be overlooked is the concern amongst carers, particularly nurses, about the growing risks from the increased incidence of AIDS. This concern is emerging as having a high correlation with stress, which in itself indicates the need for continued education, support and good administration for staff involved (Plant *et al.*, 1992).

PROVISION FOR ALCOHOLICS AND DRUG ABUSERS

Again the sufferer here may be alienated from family and friends, and by the fears of society at large. Part of the sadness for many of the victims is that they may well have suffered instability, deprivation or abuse in their own childhood and family history. They are frequently people who are held to be at the 'bottom of the pile' by self-respecting citizens and therefore they attract judgmentalism and are often accused of bringing the situation upon themselves. There is also considerable evidence of a stress-related factor, particularly for healthcare professionals (Plant *et al.*, 1992). Thus much of the provision required is as already described for other alienated individuals.

Their behaviour patterns and the friends they associate with have created anger and rejection among their family circles, particularly where they engage in criminal activities to support their addiction. Therefore any care provided needs to re-establish a sense of being valued and respected by someone who cares for them and accepts their past and present condition. Often the provision of care is exceptionally demanding over a long period of time and can only be effective where a long and trusting relationship is established. Acceptance is prepared to accept failure and disappointment and to value each person for what they are, what they can give and what they may become.

Frequently, these individuals are met with in the ordinary run of hospital or community care, where the attitudes of acceptance and trust already outlined are important. Much of the care needed, however, will be found in special clinics and residential units or through local support agencies, support groups or counsellors. Special practical social help and debt counselling may also be necessary because of the high incidence of unemployment associated with these problems. It is important that the willingness to help is continued as the patient goes on to try to rebuild a new lifestyle and also to stay by those who may never achieve this rehabilitation. These people need just as much understanding and care as anyone else and, because of their low self-esteem, can make particular demands on the carer where all attempts to help are rejected or thrown back in the face.

SPIRITUAL CARE DURING REHABILITATION AND RECOVERY

Attention inevitably tends to focus on the traumatic areas of suffering, death and bereavement, while the reality of life today is that most patients recover and return to full health or to recovery and active life even if full recovery is not achieved. It is tempting therefore to concentrate on aspects of care during the more dramatic and acute phases whereas spiritual need, care and development are part of an ongoing process of growth, response and adaptation, and are relevant to all.

Full recovery may simply mean a return to a familiar lifestyle for many but, for others, the experience of illness brings a review of life and priorities, and a search for new meaning. Some also struggle with guilt as they recover and others around them do not. This is sometimes powerfully evident in those who recover after an accident in which others die or are left incapacitated. Rehabilitation also allows a continuation of spiritual care as the process of recovery goes on over a period of time allowing an ongoing therapeutic relationship to be built (Clifford and Grucca, 1987). Staff also have more opportunity for involving families and friends as the patient is helped to respond to healing processes and with the reality of returning to full life or adapting to limited capacity.

The processes of recovery and rehabilitation have many different strands. Those severely affected by head or spinal injuries or by major trauma to the body have to face an uphill struggle in rehabilitation. They may have to relearn from scratch many daily living activities they have previously taken for granted. Alongside this is the constant pain as they go through the process and challenge of re-establishing mental and physical capacity, frequently with the knowledge that this will determine their capability for future work and social life.

So this can be a time of real challenge, grappling with frustration and disappointment and finding that things are not going as quickly as they would like. It is a time of coming to terms with accepting things that are within reach and, also, consequent limitations. This is a time when there is a need for pain to be expressed, heard and accepted; a time for realistic encouragement to stretch as far as possible and to provide incentives to keep up the effort. It is essential that professionals and family hold the balance of hope and realism and know and accept when the limits have been reached.

> *Jonathan Livingstone Seagull was an ordinary seagull who was frustrated by all his limitations and went to extraordinary lengths to overcome these.*
> *The trick – was for Jonathan to stop seeing himself as trapped inside a limited body that had a forty-two inch wing span and performance that could be plotted on a chart. The trick was to know that his true nature lived as perfect as an unwritten number, everywhere at once across space and time.*
>
> Richard Bach – *Jonathan Livingstone Seagull*

There are also moments of joy and pleasure to be recognised and shared, establishing independence in various forms and registering achievements, however small: being able to walk a few more steps; to feed; to deal with personal hygiene alone; to get back to the family. For some there is the joy of complete rehabilitation and the challenge to embrace life fully again with confidence in all its forms.

There are those for whom illness brings great debility, a need to accept the process of regaining strength for the future and to accept the need for a time of rehabilitation. This time of waiting to get back to full activity may be difficult to accept. This often follows accidents or surgery when in the recovery time there may come a period of weakness, blackness and depression. There may be a period of feeling cut-off from normal life which may lead to resentment and irritation at the attempts of friends or family who support the advice given.

There is a tendency for strong support to be given during the stages of acute illness and trauma and for it to tail away during the rehabilitation and recovery phase. In this long and slow period, there is need for continued spiritual care. Someone should be available to offer support and to be there for the patient and family to enable them to give support to one another during the process of rehabilitation where fluctuating emotions moving between elation and depression, fear and sadness, and happiness and despair may be evident and difficult to cope with.

Staff need to be available with time to listen not only to the patient but also to the family. They need to be sensitive to the opportune moment when they can enable the family to be supportive to the patient, to encourage without nagging or becoming despondent and to give confidence that, although recovery may be slow, things are proceeding normally. There is often a need to show and to encourage the ability to stand by patiently as they watch their relative struggle, without taking over in order to encourage independence. The family may also need to express their uncertainties and fears when progress is slow. Good communication is essential if the family is to work in partnership with the professionals in rehabilitation and to understand the reasons why, at some stages, it is necessary to steady the pace and at others to encourage greater efforts.

So the professionals need to build in time for these aspects of spiritual care for the person. This requires constant awareness and sensitivity to spot the moments when greater effort is needed.

This is a very difficult balance for staff to hold when their prime *raison d'etre* is to rehabilitate the person. It may be hard to accept and understand the feelings of frustration and to empathise with the moments of weakness and exhaustion. It can be a real challenge to those involved but it may be particularly hard to accept the situation when the patient decides the limit has been reached and is unwilling to struggle any further for the moment. This can be difficult when it is necessary to accept a lower standard of mobility and quality of life than that envisaged by the therapist. It can be doubly threatening when indicative that the patient has no more motivation for living.

There is a terrible agony in watching someone hollowed out with
a knife even if the end result is an instrument on which is
played the music of the universe.

Sheila Cassidy – *Good Friday People*

It is important to allow those patients who so wish, to set their own goals: to set their own mountain tops and decide the route by which they wish to climb and how far they wish to go. As in any expedition, there are some walkers who prefer to go by the gentle slopes and take time to enjoy the route, the determined climbers may choose the most direct and demanding path, and there are others whose only aim is to reach the summit as quickly and easily as possible. Each can find fulfilment in doing the journey that they wish to do. It is sometimes difficult for those who are scalers of peaks and always determined to reach the tops, to accept that there are those who can be satisfied and fulfilled in achieving lower goals.

There are some who may argue that this sounds like a distant ideal that is hard to justify in days when there are extreme pressures on staff time and facilities. It is important to remember, however, that patient recovery rates are related to morale. Thus, a patient who feels at ease within his own limitations and pace is likely to set achievable goals, to reach them successfully and to make the most effective use of resources available. So in the long run, good-quality spiritual care is also likely to be cost-effective.

PROVISION FOR SPIRITUAL CARE IN MENTAL HEALTH AND HANDICAP

A central tenet of the approach to spiritual care throughout this book has been that good spiritual care contributes to the emotional and mental wellbeing of the individual. Therefore, it is fitting to conclude these two Chapters with a synthesis of some of the thoughts already expressed.

For many people, the idea of mental health assumes freedom from mental illness and a healthy and stable personality with a normal capacity for learning and growing through experience. The concept that provision of good spiritual care is a prerequisite for all the areas considered so far would imply that there is a general contribution to mental and emotional wellbeing.Other aspects of mental illness are specialities in their own right, however, and provision needs to be seen in that light. There are three areas we will consider:

- The provision for those with learning disability.
- The provision for those affected by depressive disorders.
- The provision for those who have long-term disorders.

There is considerable change taking place in all these areas at present, as much of the organised care moves away from institutional care to community provision. Spiritual care has to be seen in that context, but the same underlying principles are always there. These principles are that the individual needs to be valued and respected and to receive an appropriate response to their needs wherever they happen to be on their own spiritual journey.

PROVISION FOR PEOPLE WITH LEARNING DIFFICULTIES

This group includes individuals with a wide range of difficulties varying from those who are simply slow at learning to those who have major or multiple disabilities. Those who are well aware that they have limitations can feel conscious that they are different from other people. They may have experienced ridicule and feel, as a consequence, that they are less valued than others – this is particularly so for children. As in many other situations, it is important to value the person just as they are and to help them to be aware of their own worth as an individual. This can then lead to the exploration that can bring to light talents and attributes that are creative and enjoyable for the individual and family concerned. It may also identify ways in which the person affected can make a real contribution to the family or community in which they live.

The important thing is to discover what they are good at – most people have something which they enjoy – and so help them to discover they can contribute in their own special way. This ensures they become conscious of sincere respect and appreciation from those around. There is clearly a need for much stimulation, and it is vital to create an environment of success and achievement as opposed to one of failure, which can easily happen if there is direct comparison with those who do not have difficulties. Equally, there is a need for support and encouragement for families to maintain that environment of achievement, so helping them towards their greatest level of independence. (See also Males *et al.*, 1990)

It is important to remember that the person with learning difficulties is also a fully spiritual person whatever their limitations of intellectual capacity. They exist fully as a person and relate to the world around them and to other people within the full extent of their ability; they experience normal emotions too. It is important to recognise that they may have a very deep need and ability to express themselves and can easily feel frustrated when this is not recognised.

Provision needs to come from all aspects of the community with the ability to accept and accommodate these people as they are and with what they have to offer. The ideal to aim for is the fullest integration into the community as opposed to segregation or rejection. Any provision made should be carefully geared to the level of understanding of the person concerned. There is still room for change of attitudes in the community to attain the desirable level of integration and acceptance. It is vital that the acceptance is sincere and not just lip service to the concept, and this may require some education. Sincerity requires listening to and journeying with that person. It is important to recognise the place of the individual and to demonstrate this recognition for the family also. The selection and training of professional staff plays a vital part in this process if the provision is to be adequate.

Provision for those with depressive disorders

Depressive disorders may take many different forms and have different origins but, once again, the underlying principle of accepting the person wherever they are on the journey is essential to any spiritual care. This acceptance and understanding may be very difficult for some, as it is threatening to stay with someone who cannot see far beyond their own depression and feels there is no hope out there at all. Great care is necessary with the way in which any response is made. People who are already plagued with a sense of guilt at their own failure, as they are unable to function normally, are often presented with tasks to perform or are encouraged to take up some occupation to help themselves out of depression. To present such a person with something to do which they feel unable to complete, simply loads the next layer of guilt into the cycle.

This is often a time to actually relieve them of demands, pressures and expectations. Initially, it can be helpful to do something with the person and share something they can join in with, especially if it is creative. This brings a sense of achievement and success and can do much to relieve feelings of guilt as the journey is shared. Clearly, there are many different forms and origins of depression and the spiritual care offered, whether by professionals or by lay carers, takes account of the individual's situation and will be integrated with the total care given to that person. To demonstrate care through the gift of time and being with the person, by staying with them as they pass through the difficult moments, may just be the clear statement of their value and worth that is so necessary.

Provision for those with psychiatric disorders

Once again, there are so many different forms and origins that the response to spiritual need will require special attention and skill and vary for each individual. In particular, it is important to listen and to understand what each individual's needs are, and what that person is trying to communicate. It is important to avoid using any approach or language which could reinforce the problems. The basic pattern is to value each individual and respond to the person where they are at that moment in their situation.

A key element in spiritual care of the mentally ill is the demonstration of the value of the person. This is of particular importance when the patient feels of little or no worth. This is a common feeling, reflecting the fears and lack of understanding of mental illness found in many cultures. To 'stay with' and 'be with' takes on a powerful significance and may well be a first step in enabling the patient to begin to come to terms with the illness, and indeed to recognise it as such and reestablish self-esteem and hope for the future (Carson, 1980). It is particularly important for spiritual care to be integrated with and complementary to medical care and management.

Through a caring committed presence people will discover :

> That they are allowed to be themselves
> That they are loved and so are lovable
> That they have gifts
> And their lives have meaning
> That they can grow and do beautiful things
> And in turn be peacemakers in a world of conflict.

Jean Vanier – *Staying*

QUESTION 1
(a) The process of rehabilitation and recovery may be long and tiring for both patients and families. Outline some of the difficulties which may be encountered. Look at the particular spiritual needs involved, discussing the challenges for the provision of good spiritual care and ways in which this can be met.
(b) Repeat question 1(a) with particular reference to mental illness or mental handicap.

QUESTION 2
Consider the effects of cultural influences and attitudes within society towards provision of long-term care for any of the groups discussed in this Chapter. Now identify ways in which the provision of good spiritual care can meet these challenges.

Key points

- Provision for long-stay patients is often overlooked but is important for the quality of care.
- This is particularly so for the elderly or physically disadvantaged, and for terminally ill patients.
- It is equally important to maintain provision for spiritual care in the community as for other types of care.
- The particular needs of AIDS and HIV sufferers should be recognised.
- Alcohol and drug abusers and their families need spiritual care, not condemnation.
- Rehabilitation and recovery are also periods often overlooked and can be times of real need for patients, families and staff.
- Special provision is needed for some aspects of mental illness and for those who have learning disabilities.
- Spiritual care has an important place in contributing to mental health and wellbeing.

CHAPTER 14

Meeting spiritual needs in different denominations or faiths

Your daily life is your temple and your religion,
Whenever you enter into it, take with you your all –
And take with you all men.

Kahlil Gibran – *The Prophet*

Just for a moment, take a step backwards in time to about 30 years ago. It is a Sunday evening, about 5.30pm, visitors have all left the ward and most patients are neatly tucked into bed awaiting their supper. The ward door opens and a small group of eager-looking individuals bursts in carrying a rickety harmonium – a signal for some of the patients who have been in for a few weeks to slide furtively under the bedclothes and start to snore gently, while others look apprehensive or bored. It is time for the 'Sunday service'. A few patients may heartily joint in singing old favourites and welcome the cheerful ministrations of the visitors. Others feel them to be totally out of place and register cool indifference or polite acceptance. Next Sunday may be the turn of the young folks guitar group or the formality of the Church ritual – all tastes have been catered for in turn.

Most of the patients will have indicated their allegiance as Church of England or perhaps as Roman Catholic, Methodist or Baptist; in some areas there will have been a small sprinkling of Jews or Muslims, but then that was probably what was expected of them – to conform to a named or an established group. As far as the hospital authorities were concerned, their spiritual needs had been catered for by a variety of worship services and 'spiritual care' had been given.

That was about 30 years ago, however, and today things have changed dramatically. That small excursion into the past may help to highlight the principles behind our provision of spiritual care today.

In terms of specific provision for formal worship, there is likely to be a variety of services broadcast over the hospital radio, local radio or television in the day room so that patients can exercise an individual choice. They may choose to listen to some form of worship in their own language or faith or not to listen at all. Patients who choose to do so, can be escorted to a live service in the hospital chapel, or can even be wheeled there in their beds. The hospital chapel may be open any time and provide a restful and quiet place where those who wish to do so can sit in peace to pray or think, or perhaps find someone to talk with.

There is now a very different perspective on what is involved in spiritual care that recognises formal worship as only one aspect of that care, and while that is indispensable to some people, it is meaningless to others.

Today we live in a multicultural society with many families, individuals and groups from a wide range of ethnic origins. Those who arrive in our care will be representative of that mixed population and we live in a multi-faith society. Even so, it does not follow that because a patient comes from a certain ethnic origin they will automatically be a practising member of a particular faith. Some may wish to maintain their religious practices, which are important to them, while others express only a nominal allegiance and are not concerned with orthodox practice at all.

SPIRITUAL CARE IN A MULTI-FAITH SOCIETY

This Chapter will look at some of the issues arising out of this multi-cultural and multi-faith society that can make good spiritual care very complex, and examples of some of the challenges will be given. Details of some specific practices and rituals that are an important aspect of care are well documented in other texts and references can be consulted (McGilloway and Myco, 1985; Neuberger, 1987).

Knowledge breeds understanding and leads to respect. Lack of knowledge often creates bigotry and projections which are wildly at variance with the truth. It is important to encourage carers in this type of mixed society to take time to learn about and to understand not just the practices but why certain practices are carried out. Without the latter, we are left with merely a one-dimensional picture. We need to know the basis of their origin and what makes them so important to members of that culture or faith.

> *Who can separate his faith from his actions,*
> *or his belief from his occupation?*
>
> Kahlil Gibran – *The Prophet*

This clearly moves a long way from the provision of a 'monochrome' and very limited response in the form of a ward service imposed on a captive audience. There the expectations were that all patients should adapt themselves to whatever was offered, rather than those who were ministering finding out what was most appropriate for the individuals concerned. Indeed, for people who were subjected to this approach and had no opportunity to remove themselves, it could be regarded as a form of mental assault.

When expanding on the need to have a regard for and an understanding of different cultures and religions, there are variations because other faiths, as well as the Christian faith, are often subdivided into different denominations. This is further complicated by individuals having their own particular view and interpretation of faith and culture. Carers need to have an overall understanding of each faith and then to apply that knowledge in the light of where each individual stands in relation to their faith or culture. They can then be sensitive to the many variations in personal tastes and needs and aim to provide the patient with whatever is most supportive and helpful at a time when religious practices, if there are any, could be vital.

Increasingly, for many whose background can be regarded as belonging to an ethnic minority group, growing up in a western culture means they frequently sit in a transcultural situation. This can be a complicated area for spiritual care as different generations within one family may have different perspectives and very different needs. The example quoted on page 00 illustrates this situation very clearly

Providing spiritual care used to be seen as a very straightforward procedure. It was true there were many different denominations to cater for and even in a predominantly Christian society, the range of different rituals and practices between denominations could make some kind of provision offensive to some patients. Provision was made by the appointment of predominantly part-time Church of England, Roman Catholic and Free Church chaplains.

But today, we see a very complex picture emerging, which underlines the need to listen and respond in an appropriate way to each person's needs. A modern chaplaincy department will have a much wider brief, with responsibilities to staff and patients of all faiths and beliefs (*see* Chapter 17), involved in education and support services and sometimes specific bereavement services.

Patients come from a wide range of ethnic and religious backgrounds embracing different practices and beliefs. The fact that an individual has a particular nationality, however, does not always mean they adhere to the predominant religion of that society. They may be orthodox and practising their traditional faith, or nominal in their adherence, or they may have embraced a different faith.

For example, an orthodox Jew may be meticulous in observing Jewish rituals and feast days, whereas some who are born as Jews may have adopted a different faith or indeed make no particular profession of faith at all.

In some societies where there is one predominant religion, this may influence the entire social structure including class differences (e.g. Hinduism and the caste system) and cultural roles (e.g. women in Muslim societies). Here individuals may adhere to local customs and traditions apparently without any particular religious reason. They may follow local customs affecting dietary patterns, or the roles of women in the family and society because that is how they have grown up. This is true of all cultures and faiths.

These factors may not all be evident when taking a history which calls for great sensitivity on the part of the carer to assess what really matters to the patient and family. It also calls for a constant readiness for staff to increase their knowledge base, to aid in understanding the reasons why certain practices prevail. Here are two examples which may help to illustrate these points.

Example

In most eastern faiths, the right hand is considered clean and the left hand unclean. In situations where there is no soap or proper cleansing facilities, the left hand is always used for cleansing the body and the right hand is used for eating and this procedure is adopted as a cultural/faith practice. This may cause problems where the right hand is injured or affected by stroke, and the patient refuses to eat with the left hand. Understanding is helped here by seeing that the custom has its origins in the simple practice of good hygiene.

Similar examples can be seen in origins of certain Jewish rituals as expounded in Old Testament law and still practised among orthodox Jews. Many of the practices relating to eating, killing animals (ritual killing ensures better preservation and cleansing), for example, were all instituted for prevention of infection in a hot climate. Adherence was ensured through their incorporation into the culture of faith teaching of the day and they have remained as a integral part of practice.

Another example is where certain foods, such as pork, are prohibited because of the difficulty of keeping the meat in a hot climate.

Recognition of these situations can lead towards bringing in someone from the faith concerned to give guidance or in some circumstances, a dispensation to the patient. Alternatively, it may be feasible for members of the family to be available to help with feeding or whatever care is needed, if they are orthodox practitioners themselves. This leads us to considering the wider practical implications for the management of spiritual care.

EXERCISE 26
- This is a good opportunity to take stock of your own experience and knowledge of other faiths. One helpful exercise is to set out the range of different religions and faiths you have come across in your care.
- Describe only particular customs or practices you have met where you needed some specific knowledge to enable you to care with more sensitivity. Put your conclusions aside and pick them up again later in the Chapter.

FACTORS AFFECTING SPIRITUAL CARE

The many different practices relating to rituals which are important to patient care are documented elsewhere: they mainly relate to diet, administration of sacramental practices or rituals, washing and dressing, and protocol for last rites. The more obvious customs may involve relationships and particular roles between members of the family and different sexes. For example, it may be inappropriate for a male nurse to attend a female patient, or there may be strong prohibitions relating to treatment such as the Jehovah's Witnesses' refusal to allow blood transfusions.

All these things have implications for those concerned with offering total care. No one person can be expected to be familiar with all these complex differences, but there should be access to information or to someone who can give more information. It is often possible to find out relevant details from the family, if there is no language problem.

Again assumptions cannot be made on the grounds of ethnic origin. There are different sects within major religions; this fact may have important consequences. In Northern Ireland, for example, a strongly Christian country is divided between Catholics and Protestants. This division is deepened by historical and political factors. This needs to be taken into account when caring for members of that society.

Failure to be aware of these differences can cause considerable distress for someone who needs the familiarity of supportive relationships and practices during a time of illness, or someone who feels unable or scared to voice personal needs or desires, or simply too ill to care very much. There are those for whom symbolism is very important and a crucifix, icon or other symbol may be of great comfort; others may appreciate someone to sit and read to them from a book of their own faith. Here the family or relatives have an important part to play in making their own customs known or even to simply say that certain practices are not vital to the person concerned. One of the main issues for carers today is to be aware of the variety of different possibilities, and to be discerning about what the individual needs and wherever possible offer real choices.

Where there are instances of specific need which are unclear, the chaplaincy or a local religious leader may be able to help with information or be able to contact someone locally who can help.

The following example illustrates the influence of western ideas on traditional practice:

A Muslim family had a stillborn child. There is no ritual in their faith for a funeral service for a child who has not lived. They were westernised in some of their ideas and particularly wanted to recognise and remember the death. They wanted to mark the death with a proper funeral. The chaplain was able to arrange and conduct an appropriate service for them. Subsequently, they had a baby born alive but who only lived a few hours. In that case the baby was able to have a Muslim funeral.

IMPLICATIONS FOR SPIRITUAL CARE: THE CARER'S APPROACH

This approach may present difficulties for some carers as they will be looking beyond their own views to enable those who have deeply held convictions about different ritual practices to be able to fulfil their own needs. Denial of that need can create real distress whereas enabling can bring a sense of peace and fulfilment.

There is often a difficulty for carers who have strongly held beliefs themselves. They may find it difficult to allow or, in particular, to assist a patient or family to carry out a practice that is contrary to their own beliefs. This is where enabling of another person to practice something contrary to one's personal beliefs needs the maturity to accept that enabling others does not mean the carer agrees with or believes in the practice, but simply accepts the right of every individual to express their own beliefs in whatever way is appropriate. The only exceptions to this would be where the practice is contrary to law, dangerous to the individual or offensive or abhorrent to others in the ward.

> *It is not always necessary that truth should find a*
> *tangible embodiment. Enough if it hovers as a spiritual essence*
> *and induces harmony by its vibrations, like the bell of*
> *solemn serenity*
>
> Goethe – in Delia Smith, *A Journey into God*

There can be dangers where those who hold fundamentalist views of any kind and see truths as absolutes have an absolute conviction that they, in their faith alone, possess knowledge of the truth and anyone who does not agree with them is automatically misguided or wrong. There is a need here for true humility to accept that what we believe profoundly does not automatically make those beliefs the whole truth. There has to be the capacity for us as human beings to recognise that none of us holds a monopoly on the truth, and to be prepared to acknowledge we may not always be right.

If we expect to have the right not only to hold our own beliefs, but also to have them respected and to have the right to practice them, dare we offer less to others? Where a spirit of openness exists, we may be surprised at how much common ground can be established between members of different faiths and how much fellow feeling can be engendered by a willingness not only to share our own beliefs, but also to listen to those of other faiths. There is a very deep rapport that can be established which gives the opportunity to support at a deep level those going through spiritual pain. This comes only from mutual respect, understanding and willingness to enable that individual to express themselves and their feelings not just in words, but also in the practice of their faith and culture. There are very important ethical principles involved here which need to be thought through carefully.

> Our highest truths are but half truths.
> Think not to settle down for ever in any truth
> Make use of it as a tent in which to pass a summer's night
> But build no house of it, or it will be your tomb.
> When you first have an inkling of its insufficiency
> And begin to descry a dim counter truth looming up beyond,
> Then weep not, but give thanks,
> It is the Lord's voice whispering: 'Take up thy bed and walk'

J J Balfour – in *The Bridge of Love*, Bishop of Stockwood

Identification of religious needs is thus one very important aspect of spiritual care needing particular recognition during the assessment stages of care. Considerable sensitivity is required from carers in the early days after admission. The patient may be totally unaware of the significance of some of the issues involved and so may not reveal his beliefs until the need arises and the trust has been established with the care given.

Nurses are perhaps more likely to meet up with these implications than others in the team as they provide a more continuous service over the 24-hour span. No one professional carer will be completely aware of all the complexities and, for this reason, good communication within the team and a willingness to share care with other team members is essential, together with a known resource where further information and help can be sought.

Sometimes patients say they have no religion – they are agnostics, atheists, humanists or pagan for example and so may be thought to have no specific religious requirements. This highlights the importance of asking appropriate questions on admission because many of these people will have thought through the issues concerned and made a conscious decision about their belief and value systems. They will still need to find meaning in the experiences encountered, however, and in the way they respond (Burnard, 1988). They may also have other specific wishes, for example, pagans like to know when death is impending and to have time to make their own preparations (Prout, 1992).

Some aspects of care need particular attention and carers need to be familiar with normal practices for the major religions including facilities for worship, prayer and the sacraments, special dietary requirements, rituals to mark birth or transitions to adulthood, care during dying and procedure after death including funeral arrangements. For some religious groups, such as Jehovah's Witnesses, there are strong objections to blood transfusions or to organ transplants and others such as Christian Scientists will not consent to organ donation. Detailed practical aspects relating to these issues can be found elsewhere (Neuberger, 1987; Green, 1991).

EXERCISE 28

This is a point at which you may be ready to examine some of your own beliefs. Look at some practices related to religious care, and indicate where you find difficulty in accepting these and why. Go on to discuss in your group ways in which you manage to overcome these difficulties, and recognise any area of prejudice.

Reference to transcultural influences was made earlier and the following example shows how it is possible to offer a sympathetic caring approach to a complex situation:

Example

Different generations may hold differing views within their own faiths, particularly where the second generation has grown up in a different cultural milieu. A young Indian couple had a stillborn child and the medical staff wished to perform a postmortem examination. The family as a whole held strong traditional views that the body should not in any way be mutilated after death and that there should be an early funeral.

The young couple, however, had grown up and been educated into western culture and, while wishing to observe the funeral ritual of the Hindu faith, also recognised the value and importance for their own family future of having a postmortem carried out. This was resolved without offence to the larger family by the couple agreeing to the postmortem in discussion when the rest of the family were not present and so not offended in any way. The necessary genetic counselling was then made possible in the light of information gained.

As already indicated, there are other less well known practices relating to sacred garments, symbolic articles or the use of touch. It helps considerably if the carer knows something about the basic beliefs and philosophies of the various religions concerned. It also helps if they are prepared to consider their own approach to questions about the value of the individual and if they are aware of their own attitudes and beliefs relating to life-and death-issues. It is also important to set these aspects of religious care in the total context of the whole spectrum of spiritual care, which makes such a valuable contribution to the patient's general comfort, wellbeing and recovery. It is also important to ask patients and their families what their needs are.

EXERCISE 29
Look back at your conclusions to the previous two exercises and set out the areas where you have gaps in your knowledge or experience and would like to explore the subject further.

QUESTION I
References to specific further reading at the end of the book will assist with your answers.
(a) Summarise the aspects of healthcare in which you think all professionals need a basic knowledge of the spiritual care and religious needs of a range of ethics and cultural groups. Which of these is particularly relevant to your own professional practice?
(b) Describe a patient or family you have cared for where religious needs posed a particular challenge and say how this challenge was approached. Would you now make any modifications to the care offered? Make reference to any literature you have read.

Key points

- Changing perspectives towards spiritual care mean that there is likely to be a range of options available today to assist patients from different faiths and cultures to worship.
- There is a need for carers to understand different cultures and religions, and to recognise the variations that exist.
- Recognition of these differences calls for great sensitivity on the part of carers assessing needs.
- This presents a challenge to carers to look beyond their own beliefs and to respect the rights of others to practice according to their conscience.
- Some practical aspects of care will need particular attention where patients and families have special needs to be respected.

CHAPTER 15

Special needs in controversial situations: dilemmas and decisions

Where is the life we have lost in living?
Where is the wisdom we have lost in knowledge?
Where is the knowledge we have lost in information?

TS Eliot – *The Four Quartets*

The complexities surrounding ethical issues arising during caring for individuals in sickness or in health have never been more prominent than they are today. The media and press coverage ensure that the general public are alerted to many of the situations arising, and therefore they want to have questions answered about the issues raised.

THE CURRENT PERSPECTIVE

A major complication today is the speed at which change is taking place. There is ever-changing medical knowledge and development of new drugs and surgical techniques. In addition, there is increasing use of new technology to take over more and more bodily functions. All these pose questions which are important to those involved including the patient, relatives and carers. Any new treatments have implications for all of these groups.

The days are gone when carers used all known treatments available until they ran out, when death would occur. This simplistic situation no longer occurs in the developed world. Medical knowledge and the range of treatments and surgery now available continues to escalate. This has brought a number of important ethical questions into focus; for example, questions relating to when it is right to use or to withhold the use of life-support systems, whether life-support systems should be continued or discontinued, and upon what criteria should such decisions and judgments can be made.

Other dilemmas occur concerning the timing of movement from critical or curative care to palliative or terminal care. These questions relating to the timing of intervention are clearly more easily solved if there is time to look carefully and openly at all options and the implications involved. It helps if there is opportunity to discuss these issues with the patient, family and amongst professionals, with access to all information available. More difficult situations arise where swift decisions have to be made in the middle of a crisis, either on admission to hospital or when a particular problem arises unexpectedly.

In crisis moments it sometimes happens that the person or people faced with making an 'on-the-spot' decision do not always have sufficient experience to justify the decision taken or to see the full implications, whereas a more experienced person could use their knowledge and wisdom to avoid prolonging existence unnecessarily.

Clearly any such decision not to begin an intervention which is available can lead to strong responses from the patient, relatives or staff. This is particularly true where staff members have strong principles relating to preservation of life being pre-eminent and must be attempted at all costs This brings a corollary that it is always wrong to refuse treatment to anyone at any time. Such situations can give rise to considerable tensions and pressure for staff.

MAKING CHOICES – CRITERIA INVOLVED

> *When you have to make a choice, and don't make it, that is in itself a choice.*
> William James – In Delia Smith, *Journey into God*

It is thus apparent that the rapid growth of technological change has left the human race to face an ever widening range of possibilities for improvement, with difficult choices to make. There can be several choices, some involving moral issues, where each one seems to be equally unacceptable and any one ultimately selected involves a painful decision.

Example
A classic example often quoted is a situation where a father is faced with a violent intruder threatening to kill his wife and family. The father, a peace-loving man, has to decide whether to attack him or to see his wife and children die. Hostage-taking is another example. There are many situations where we are faced with two evils, both involving painful choices with consequent emotional trauma, spiritual guilt and pain.

Making choices can involve a whole range of criteria on which to draw and base decisions, many of which are discussed in this Chapter. Criteria include the ethical and moral principles of all those involved, and may be influenced by cultural and religious background, so every decision becomes a complex situation depending on many variables. What may be best for one may be totally unacceptable to another.

Sometimes there is a knowledge base to inform and assist in making decisions, but the resources to act are unavailable. This kind of decision increasingly faces those in the caring professions these days. If resources are inadequate to provide patients with safe and proper care, the question is whether you keep a ward open and struggle on with minimal care risking dangerous practice, or close the ward and risk people having to wait for treatment or indeed to die prematurely. The healthcare professionals are one of the groups who most often come face to face with controversial and painful situations of this kind in their work situations. Some of these involve life-and-death dilemmas, while others relate to the quality of life.

Other decisions may have a topical or seasonal nature, as at the present time, when debate ranges around resources available and what the alternatives are. One example is in the controversy between doctors in some centres who will not undertake major heart surgery on patients who will not give up smoking, and those who consider all should be treated equally and have access to surgery irrespective of lifestyle. Criteria in this area involve the knowledge of the detrimental effects of smoking on the health of patients and others and the technology available together with the chances of treatment being successful, all set in the context of the resources available and the principle of universality of access to treatment.

Clearly the possible outcomes can be backed up by research findings in such a case, but there are value judgments to be made and many parallel situations can be ignored in the light of heated discussion. Consider the point that most of us in some way or another have a lifestyle which may damage our health or physical capacity, maybe through ignorance or poverty or sheer self-indulgence. We may drink excessively, over-eat or fail to eat a balanced diet or to take enough exercise or sleep – so where should the line be drawn? Is it right to give treatment only to the deserving? Some would argue that everyone should have the right to be treated. Then we face the problem of limited resources, however, what basis the allocation should be made and where the use of resources will create the most beneficial outcome?

There are always counter-balancing factors and taking such arguments further down the line leads us into the realm of wide-ranging criteria. Take a heavy smoker aged 40 years with a dependent wife and several children to support and set this against a non-smoking and non-drinking person aged 70 with no dependents. What weight should be given to the various aspects of the argument when taxpayers' money and insurance is involved? On what grounds can treatment be denied, or how heavily are the criteria arguments to be weighted?

Using the age of the person as a general criterion can be a very blunt instrument because many other criteria make the projected outcome variable and individual. Often there are no specific answers to give and many differing views to consider and the solution for one case is totally impracticable for another. There are also many people involved: the patient, the family and the professionals who give the care, and often the management authorities, legal advisers or general public and politicians. This is thus a subject of enormous complexity with no easy answers to be given – particularly in the space of one Chapter!

We will not attempt to explore in depth the fundamental ethics involved in all these cases as that is well documented by other writers (Rumbold, 1986; Tschudin, 1992). All that is possible here is to look at some of the underlying principles involved in meeting and providing spiritual need and care in such situations, and suggest how carers and sufferers can be best helped to find their way through the labyrinth and perhaps to give a few examples from current debate.

FACTORS CAUSING THE DILEMMA

Behind most values and beliefs in the medical and nursing professions, there is a fundamental belief in the value of each human life, regardless of colour, creed or any other differences as seen, for example, in the Hippocratic oath or in the International Code of Nursing Ethics (1992). The basic principle is one of valuing each life irrespective of lifestyle, and part of this principle is about doing nothing harmful to the patient. For example, a tramp arriving in accident and emergency unit with a fractured femur is given the same kind of treatment and respect as an elite athlete or famous golfer. Inherent in all medical and professional codes of practice is the understanding and acceptance that judgmental attitudes will be avoided. These principles are coming increasingly under threat with current financial pressures. They are being evaluated afresh in the light of limited resources and also projected outcome now comes into the ethical considerations used in order to make the best use of the resources available.

THE DILEMMA OF LIMITED RESOURCES

As we look at other examples where decisions are complicated, we see many relate to situations where limited resources are key criteria. In some cases, there are arguments on both sides. The current limited availability of more advanced treatments for infertility is a case in point. There is no life-threatening situation involved and there is a matter of choice involved because there are options such as adoption or fostering which could be considered as alternatives. On the other side, almost all reasons for infertility are the result of disease or bodily malfunction such as endometriosis, emotile sperm, or low sperm count. While a range of treatments for infertility is available through the NHS, in-vitro fertilisation is not.

There are ethical dilemmas associated with in-vitro fertilisation where there are no dimensions of life-threatening implications or indeed where there is no physical pain or debility involved. Nevertheless, there are incorporated areas of deep suffering and feelings of deprivation and lack of personal fulfilment in life.

Thus, there is an uneasy and difficult line drawn between the range of treatments given under the NHS and that which is available privately and most treatment for in-vitro fertilisation, for example, is given privately at present.

The question of limited resources is one of the most painful areas for ethical debate and its assessment affects our decision making in healthcare and the identification of the criteria to be used for allocation. At present these issues are not fully resolved and clearly there are many conflicting opinions. Another obvious example is seen in the treatment of HIV-positive and AIDS patients, which is an area where it has been accepted every treatment area must be comparatively well resourced, despite the fact that certain lifestyles clearly make some groups more exposed to risk. This all conflicts with the stance, taken in some centres, where treatment is withheld to smokers.

The pressures come in particular to those who have limited resources in terms of finance, personnel, expertise and time available. If there are 100 people needing treatment and only facilities available for 75, some kind of selective criteria will have to be applied. Part of the argument with smoking and lung cancer is about short-term recovery chances and anaesthetic risks, but there is yet a further set of questions about future lifestyle and its possible consequences for further treatment or intervention at a later stage.

DIFFERENT PERSPECTIVES

The needs of staff may be different from the needs of the relatives or the patient, as they all have a different perspective on the situation. The patient may be governed by what he feels about the likely outcome of a decision and that may override a rational decision or lead to acceptance of something which would normally go against personal principles. The family may see it very differently; for example, where a question of terminating pregnancy is involved perhaps where there is a possibility of a malformed baby. Here the mother may be totally unable to accept the possibility of such a future but the family may have strongly held religious principles and be horrified about such an action.

The professional staff could well have yet another perspective as they have a knowledge base from which to decide, and the mother's future health and wellbeing could be seriously threatened. Such an example clearly shows the need for good communication, shared discussion and support of each individual related to their own personal needs.

There are also political and social perspectives involved with making choices. A recent editorial (Dimond, 1993) explores the question of 'Who deserves care?' and looks at the case relating to a range of different groups including single parents, people who have attempted suicide, people with sports injuries, the elderly, mentally infirm and reckless drivers. The writer asks whether they are entitled to care or treatment in a cash-restricted society and concludes 'There are few who can be said to deserve care but many who need it.'

ETHICAL PRINCIPLES RELEVANT TO PROVISION OF SPIRITUAL CARE

Throughout this text words have been used repeatedly that may have different meanings for many of us, yet they are all implicit in the principles governing what we do each day. They are words such as 'beliefs, values, judgments, rights, responsibilities, good, quality of life, the meaning of life ...' and so on. So how can we establish some basic guidelines to help staff who find the modern dilemmas so pressurising and to help the patient and family who are often faced with decisions equipped with limited knowledge and with strong personal and emotional agendas which may cloud the picture?

Most of us behave in fairly predictable ways every day without necessarily stopping to ask why we behave as we do. Indeed, if we did that too often we would end up like the proverbial centipede – in the ditch! When it comes to issues that relate to the major traumas of life and death, however, a range of unwelcome options are often presented and we find then that there are a number of factors that govern our decisions.

As individuals we have our own cultural and religious background where strongly held convictions or beliefs may help or hinder making decisions and may sometimes actually remove any element of choice. Sometimes legal implications influence us or political motives prompt us to act a certain way. It may be that we act intuitively in response to events or that conscience dictates how we behave. It is likely that many healthcare staff will be very strongly motivated by a deep rooted desire to care. We may not be crystal clear about how these motives affect our behaviour in the event of a situation which challenges our own perspectives. Strong feelings may arise, however, presenting a painful dilemma where anger, resentment or aggressive responses may erupt.

EXERCISE 30

Individual carers can prepare for situations which arise to some extent by sorting out for themselves what they actually believe, what motivates them and what values are common to most of us. (Some of these issues may have been sorted out already from previous exercises. The questions can be dealt with on your own or with others in a group.)
- How do I decide what is a 'right' course of action in a situation?
- Do I rely on my beliefs, my 'conscience', my intuitive feelings or my relevant professional knowledge?
- Think of a recent situation in your experience and explore how it looks from each of the above points of view.

When it comes to professional practice, we start with our own convictions and perspectives, but there is also the additional guide for most of us to be found in our own Code of Professional Practice. Each profession will have slight variations in general principles but, basically, a code protects the patient from any malpractice and also protects the practitioner by giving general principles or guidelines to practice. In addition to this, there is a recognised base of knowledge from which the carer can start.

All of this, however, has to be relevant to day-to-day practice and may be inadequate when it comes to the way in which we face life-and-death issues. Most patients and families do not have some of these guides to help them and may be thrown back onto public opinion and the media for assistance. They might therefore feel very threatened and look to the professionals for straight answers where none exist.

The dilemma may not be one that requires a sudden dramatic decision. Often it is a situation which has evolved over a number of years and involves close family relationships. This is increasingly so as more families are faced with caring for the elderly or mentally sick in the community.

Example

Kathy was in her eighties having lived independently since her husband died 10 years ago. Her daughter, Jane, and family lived about 15 miles away and visited with their children every few weeks. They never had very close relationships and Kathy was often very disapproving of the way they were handling the children, now growing into their teens. Her health was now failing, however, and after several spells in hospital it became evident she needed help. Peter and Jane felt responsible and although their home was rather cramped decided Kathy should move in with them.

It was soon evident that this was causing severe disruption to their family life. The children felt their freedom was restricted and became embarrassed to bring friends home and so started staying out late, which caused constant rows in the family. Relationships between Peter and Jane were reaching breaking point and Kathy was beginning to feel unwanted and rejected.

This is a common enough situation these days, but one causing an ethical dilemma as well as a practical one for the family, the patient and the professional carers. It is also a political and social dilemma. Thus, on all counts, it presents a challenge in terms of spiritual care, when so often everyone is caught up in the practical issues and ready to say what 'ought to be done' in a prescriptive manner.

Many ethical situations, however, are much more dramatic in their presentation and therefore tend to receive more publicity as in the issues surrounding abortion, euthanasia, withdrawing life support, or a whole range of dilemmas surrounding donor transplants. Such issues are frequently under scrutiny in the media by politicians, professionals and religious leaders. The debates tend to intensify from time to time as views change with current fashions or some new discovery or when some major incident focuses attention on the subject for a while.

EXERCISE 31

Look again at the example described above. Take this as a practical situation for a care review, among professionals; and consider it with particular reference to the spiritual care of:
- Kathy
- The family.

Look at the range of options open to them and consider the implications of any decisions made. What spiritual care is needed in each case and who is involved in the team approach? This is a situation with far-reaching implications either way and a good comprehensive issue to help in sorting out the best care plan for all concerned.

ETHICAL CORE OF SPIRITUAL CARE

Most people would like to have some firm guidelines to follow as we all feel threatened and inadequate when faced with so many options and choices. Usually, it is not possible to offer definitive answers to such complex questions and each situation has to be assessed in the light of the current knowledge, the rights and needs of the individual concerned, and resources available. The kind of questions raised have no clear answers: 'What is the right thing to do? What is best for the individual? What are the choices and which of them will cause the least harm?'.

It is always useful to have thought through possible options beforehand, however, and then a more informed decision can be made on the basis of the particular situation presented. Consideration of principles involves personal views and preferences, and also the need to recognise what the community at large can accept. This may prove complicated in a multi-faith and multi-cultural society where basic morals are difficult to identify.

While there are no clear-cut rules applicable in all cases, there are some basic principles which can help in making some of these complex decisions. One important principle, for example, is the need to recognise the rights of the individual to be consulted about treatment offered and, in so far as is possible, to be guided by decisions which they in all conscience believe to be right. Difficulties arise here where a child or unconscious patient is involved. For example, adult Jehovah's Witnesses may refuse blood transfusions themselves, but where their child is concerned the principle involves a new dimension, especially in a life-threatening situation. Not all professionals can accept that it is valid to refuse such treatment to a child.

A similar guiding principle is the need to preserve the dignity of the individual at all times, allowing the patient to retain autonomy and the best quality of life possible in line with their personal preferences.

Another example of a principle essential to all practice of spiritual care is the need to maintain and respect confidentiality. This is an area that gives rise to conflict at times when the carer may feel the family or colleagues should know what has been disclosed. This principle can give rise to many uncertainties where confidential information has been shared in a counselling situation or between colleagues in a support group. It is particularly difficult where disclosures relating to issues such as drug abuse or violent tendencies are concerned.

The underlying principle is to respect confidentiality at all times except where there may be a real life-threatening situation or a threat to the safety of others where disclosure is required by law. This kind of dilemma emphasises the importance for counsellors to have access to experienced supervisors, for support groups to have access to facilitators who can give them guidance over issues like these, and for professional staff to know where they can turn for personal support themselves.

PRACTICAL GUIDELINES

To conclude this Chapter and offer some guidelines, it may be helpful to look at a few examples or questions and use these as discussion points around a principle. In facing complex issues, it is always useful to have thought through the possible options and then an informed choice or decision can be made on the basis of the situation presented. Consideration of principles involves personal opinions and requires recognition of what the community will find acceptable.

For professionals, conflict may arise because the caring relationship is basic to all their practice and a 'precondition of all cure' (Nouwen, 1987). Several writers refer to the '5 Cs of caring' (Roach, 1987; Tschudin, 1992). These are compassion, competence, confidence, commitment and conscience, which sum up a basis for all actions. These principles, however, may give rise to considerable emotional conflicts for carers and this is where they need adequate provision for support as discussed in

Chapter 18. Equally, conflicts of different kinds arise for patients, families and friends involved with the decisions, which may indicate a need for special counselling and support to be given.

QUESTION 1a
Principle: preserving the right of the individual.
The surgical team has agreed in principle that blood will not be given to a Jehovah's Witness during operation. An emergency arises unexpectedly, however, and to withhold blood would be fatal so the team decides to give blood on the basis that the patient is unconscious and unable to decide.

QUESTION 1b
If you were leading the surgical team, would you sanction giving blood? Justify your decision.

QUESTION 2
Principle: the right to discontinue treatment.
(a) Is it ethical to continue giving painful treatment causing acute discomfort when it is known that it cannot improve the length or quality of life?
(b) Who should make the decision to discontinue – the patient, relatives or professionals?
(c) Does the patient have the right to refuse treatment that can be beneficial and, if so, under what circumstances?
(d) What do you consider to be the key factor in these issues?

QUESTION 3
Principle: preservation of life.
(a) Should life be preserved at all costs?
(b) Is it ethical to make judgments on the basis of inadequate resources and what criteria should be applied?

QUESTION 4
Principle: all patients should have equal access to treatment and resources should be fairly divided
(a) What is 'equality of care'?
(b) Do you deny treatment to a handicapped child and give it to an athlete on the basis that he is a potential medallist, or do you give it to the child on the basis that he is already underprivileged?
Some useful questions to consider to guide your discussion might include:
• Will this course of action result in the good of this patient?
• Does the course of action relieve pain and suffering?

- Does is create more suffering?
- Is the treatment more damaging than the condition?
- Does it improve the quality of life?

QUESTION 5
Think back over the work you have done on this Chapter. Outline your own personal values and beliefs which you find are useful in making ethical decisions.

QUESTION 6
Confidentiality is an issue assuming greater importance these days. Discuss some of the ethical issues which may cause difficulties between:(a) Families, patients and professionals. (b) Carers in different professions, and colleagues.
Indicate some of the courses of action you have followed and identify the principles which guided you in your actions.

QUESTION 7
Do you think all patients have a right to have access to full medical treatment and care regardless of age, lifestyle and other circumstances? Discuss some of the issues involved in arriving at your conclusions looking at the arguments from the perspectives of the patient, the family and the professionals.

Key points

- The current scenario has accelerated the rate of change in healthcare situations and created complex ethical dilemmas for carers.
- Often there are many conflicting factors to consider and a range of criteria involved.
- Decisions have to be made in the context of limited resources. Political and social perspectives are involved and, in addition, issues are complicated by media attention.
- There are no clear-cut answers, but carers may refer to some basic principles to help them arrive at decisions.

Section V

Practical issues in management and delivery of spiritual care

Provision for particular needs, as we have seen in the previous Section, is essential for establishing a framework for meeting spiritual needs. There is one element which needs special consideration – the caring team – as the quality of care is dependent on the staff who have a major role in the communication and delivery of care.

With that in mind, this Section concentrates on the caring team, building on some of the areas identified in Section II in relation to skills and individual strengths. Preparation for giving care will be explored, together with aspects of staff support, education and the resources available. This Section brings around in full circle the various areas isolated for detailed consideration throughout this text. It brings the focus back to looking at the integration of staff resources and provision of care in the light of patient need.

CHAPTER 16

The caring team – roles, relationships and responsibilities

The symphony needs each note
The book needs each page
The house needs each brick
The ocean needs each drop of water
The harvest needs each grain of wheat –

Michael Quoist – *The Breath of Life*

The delivery of spiritual care is by no means the sole perogative of any one particular profession or individual member of staff. We bring the whole of ourselves, our skills and personalities to relate to individuals needing care, and seek to see each individual as a whole person needing care in all aspects of their lives. This kind of care requires a range of skills which may be offered by a range of different professional carers working in close liaison with the family, volunteers, friends and, most essentially, the patient himself.

Spiritual care cannot be put in a box and labelled until the right person comes along because spiritual need is there at any time during the process of treatment and recovery: the need is always there. It may be that one particular person in the team spends more time than the others with the patient, however, and thus has more opportunity to listen and identify needs. It may be that another person has the skills to meet this need or a particular affinity with a patient or family and is so able to establish the partnership relationship discussed earlier.

Just as a number of different professionals are involved with care, so there are carers at different levels of the organisation's structure. For example, the management may well be responsible for ensuring the various provisions discussed in Chapter 15 are adequate, but the staff who actually deliver the hands-on care may come in at any level of experience for different purposes.

Skill mix has become a very important aspect of management today, and there is an implicit responsibility to ensure that a range of expertise is available, that staff know their degree of responsibility, that they establish common agreed goals within an integrated care plan, and have adequate communication channels (Brill, 1976).

While each member has specific skills and a personal contribution to make, there are inevitably areas of overlap and roles can become blurred (Vachon, 1998). This is described very clearly in a Working Party Report, *Mud and Stars*, from Sir Michael Sobell House (1991), using the diagram illustrated below.

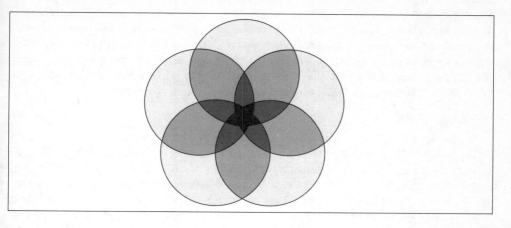

Diagram illustrating role responsibility in teamwork. Each circle represents a different profession. The shaded areas indicate the overlap in tasks and roles which occurs in teamwork. The star area in the centre indicates where all care should be integrated, i.e. the spiritual aspects of patient care.

EXERCISE 32

There is an interesting exercise you can do for yourself here – look at the diagram above for a moment then put the original to one side and reproduce it yourself. Did you manage to get it the same the first time? What were the differences between yours and the original? Many people have found it extremely difficult to do, frequently ending up with a hole in the middle instead of a heavily shaded area, as in the diagram below.

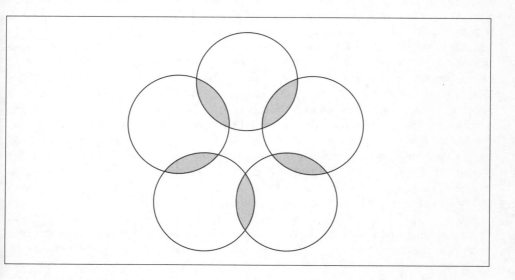

The circles represent different professions, the shaded areas indicating a measure of overlap in roles between two or more carers. It is clear, however, that there is a central area in the original diagram where every carer has a contribution to make. This could be interpreted as the area of spiritual care, in which everyone is involved. The second diagram shows what could happen where it is assumed that spiritual care is the responsibility of someone else, or if communication is not good and full implications of roles and responsibilities are not clear. Where there is good team interaction and a full awareness that everyone is involved, there is a responsibility in spiritual care accepted by all members of the team and the quality and continuity of care is assured.

The *Mud and Stars* report identifies at least 28 different professional teams or groups ranging through administrators, nurses, medical and chaplaincy teams, support teams, informal carers, therapists and volunteers. These groups may operate in hospitals or community settings, some members being involved in several different teams. It is often forgotten that at the centre of all these different teams is the patient – the one person involved throughout the process and so often not consulted!

MANAGEMENT OF SPIRITUAL CARE THROUGH TEAMWORK

It is important to recognise that the management of spiritual care is as important as other aspects of management or patient care. So often it is ignored, or dealt with piecemeal, or in a maverick way where individuals decide they have the particular skills required and shirk communication with others in the team.

Clearly matters of confidentiality can arise in this area, but can usually be managed without breaking confidences. For most people opening up the deepest areas of spiritual need is something that can best be done with one person only or at most with two to three very trusted individuals. This in itself can sometimes be a source of frustration or guilt. It may even give rise to jealousy when team members feel that the person being used in that role by the patient or family is far less skilled than themselves or that this task is their particular responsibility. All those involved in the care of the patient have some role to play in meeting spiritual needs and, as far as possible, all members of the caring team of professionals, those working in a supportive capacity and also family members have their part to play.

The pattern is similar to the medical pattern where doctors, nurses, physiotherapists, nutritionists and others all have specific roles to play. If you look within the professions, there may be more than one speciality amongst the doctors or specialist nursing staff involved in addition to the ward or community team. But to ensure that good nursing or medical care is given, all the different aspects need to be coordinated working to the accepted care plan.

So too in spiritual care it is important that everyone involved recognises the need to work towards the same aims and objectives, accepting that each has a different part to play. In particular there is a need to accept the place of the key person chosen by the patient or relative, and to recognise that if we believe in patient-centred care, the patient holds the right to choose the person with whom they feel most at ease. It is also important here to distinguish between the needs of the patient and the relative as they may be very different.

It is important to make the point here that the prime responsibility for giving continuous spiritual care inevitably lies with the nursing staff who are there all the time. They are likely to be the key people, if not always, for the in-depth care at least as facilitators of that process with the responsibility to ensure that spiritual care is given. It is important that nurses recognise and value the skills of other members of the team and bring them in and involve them wherever appropriate so that the best and most appropriate spiritual care can be given.

One more thing to recognise is that there are times when it is necessary to bring someone who is a little removed from day-to-day care into the picture more prominently. This should not be seen as a criticism of those giving the daily care, but rather as a recognition that the patient may need someone perceived to be slightly apart from decisions about their treatment or care, or someone perceived to have particular skills, attitudes or beliefs. This is an area where chaplains and social workers (although they often do have a specific role) may be able to come into the picture and facilitate some kind of exploration for the patient which may be difficult for those on the spot who are so closely involved with the day-to-day care. To share the deepest and most personal aspects of the self, the patient may need to have someone who is trusted to give absolute confidentiality (as contrasted with confidentiality in a professional role).

EXERCISE 33

Consider the range of professionals involved in spiritual care in your own workplace at present. Explore within your group the nature of their expertise and look at the various ways in which you have found them useful. Discuss examples from your group experience.
• How can you ensure full coordination of these skills in your team?
• How do you decide when to share the situation with someone else?

One of the things which may happen in the course of treatment is that a strong bond develops between the patient and nursing or medical staff. This may deter the patient from questioning decisions to terminate treatment that may be seen as life saving. The patient may feel it is not fair to open this subject with staff. This again may be difficult to explore with family or friends because of bonds existing and causing pain for those they love.

PRESSURES FOR THE TEAM

Teamwork in itself can make demands on the individual members and it creates its own stress, but it can also bring rewards in terms of learning from each other and adding strengths to the total care available. The sum total of a team's contribution is always more than the sum of the individual contributions. One strength is seen as individual members of the team share different abilities, values and experiences. This does call for good communication, however, if the spiritual needs are to be met by the most appropriate person as members need to be prepared to pass on responsibility where the need for this is apparent. Sadly, some who have strong beliefs act as if they are the only resource available and actively block others from giving spiritual care (even when it has been asked for by the patient). Shared goals and mutual dependence are important and the humility to accept that some members may be more able to cope with difficult emotional situations than others.

Confidentiality may pose a problem within the team as a patient may share something with one member of the team who feels inadequate to handle the situation, but is not sure whether it was meant to be passed on. It is helpful if the team have an understanding between themselves about the way in which these situations can be managed and also if the patient is aware of the interdisciplinary aspects of team care. There are, of course, particular advantages where the patient is fully accepted as a team member and so is involved in discussion on his care. Unfortunately, this is still not a universal situation which means an important dimension of understanding spiritual need is missing when discussions take place (Owen, 1989).

One area where the value of the team is noticeably relevant is where patients have particular religious or cultural needs and one member of the team has special understanding of that faith or culture. Sometimes one person may feel unable to cope with exploration of fears or to handle the expression of anger because of their own experiences or prejudices, and they need to feel it is acceptable to pass on the responsibility to another person. This may also be in the interests of respecting the personal needs of the staff member.

Good teamwork will undoubtedly enhance the quality of spiritual care available for patients, clients and relatives. It will also bring added strength to the members involved as they learn from each other finding opportunities for self-development and support, sharing experiences and skills in the process.

It is within the team that many staff find mutual support and understanding and grow even through situations of conflict. The next Chapter will look in more detail at ways of establishing this kind of support and other aspects of caring for staff.

QUESTION 1

(a) Is there an aspect or core of spiritual care you can identify in which every member of the caring team is involved? How do you define this and how do you ensure it is covered?

(b) How can different roles of professionals, and expectations of carers and patients affect the quality of spiritual care offered? Discuss this with reference to role theory and illustrate with practical examples from your own experience.

Key points

- Spiritual care requires a range of skills and is not the sole prerogative of any one person.
- All members of the team need to work towards the same aim and objectives in providing spiritual care.
- It is important to recognise when it is necessary to bring in other members of the team. Here confidentiality may pose a problem within the team.

Resources for spiritual care – finding and facilitating

In the area of responding to spiritual need, helplessness often arises in the carers, the patient and the family. There is a feeling of isolation, of being alone and without any tangible resources available to back up the care given, and this is a misconception. This Chapter will look separately at resources for patients and families and then for carers, although there will be some overlap.

RESOURCES FOR THE PATIENT AND FAMILY

We should remind ourselves once again of the need to recognise the existing resources already within the patient and family as that is where we need to start. These resources may be disabled by the events which have happened, but each member involved will have built up patterns of understanding, belief and response which, although temporarily disabled, can be re-activated. It is therefore important for the carer to assess the resources the family already have and use.

There are then two steps to take: first of all, to find out where the patient and family stand already, which must be the starting point. Secondly, we need to identify the needs which have not been met and so assess what further support and help can be usefully brought in. There may be a key person or group that is valued and trusted that could give continued support and care and that would maintain that relationship once there is a return to home and community life. It is equally important to listen to the patient and family, and to their patterns of response which may identify inappropriate avenues for support – avenues which may on the surface look right to the carer but are alien to the person concerned.

It is good to have a range of options or avenues in mind and to try to use them appropriately for the individual. The timing of offering help is crucial, for example, knowing just when it would be acceptable to suggest joining a support group. This could be welcome to some but not acceptable to everyone, or acceptable at a later time but not at the outset. The offer of an opportunity to meet with someone who has had a similar experience may be acceptable sometimes, but not always. These suggestions need to be made with sensitivity and at the right time if they are to be effective.

Literature or leaflets may be appreciated by some people whereas others may not want to be bothered by this or be able to use it properly – they may even be offended by it. Literature is most useful when used to establish or further an ongoing dialogue and to open the door to further discussion and exploration. It can also be used as an *aide memoire* which can be referred to when alone. Again leaflets need careful selection and must be relevant to the situation and not simply used as a means to say just what has taken place. They must provide good clear information in language that is generally understood, and be well prepared and presented.

USING VOLUNTEERS

Volunteers are an excellent resource if they are acceptable to the patient and family. It is essential that they are carefully selected for this role and prepared for the work they undertake. Their activities need regular monitoring and the volunteers themselves need good support. For many volunteers, a short training course introducing them to some of the practical skills of listening, helping and knowing where to go for assistance if needed, is useful and gives confidence. There is a danger if they are just let loose without preparation in the belief that any willing person can be helpful. This can create problems which can take more time to untangle than the time saved by their input. It is important to ensure they are not put into difficult situations they cannot handle and that there is always help available if they find themselves in deep water. The role of the volunteer is not to replace professional input or to save money, but to enhance the care given.

USING THE FAMILY GROUP

It is always important to encourage help within the family circle where it is acceptable and relationships are supportive. The family is an important resource as its members are known to each other and they can provide continuing care after discharge from hospital. They can be a useful ongoing support group, but they may well require professional support and guidance themselves from time to time, to develop their understanding of the situation, their needs, and also to give confidence in the care they are giving.

The right focus is important – the primary supporters of the person are those already there who are known and have a key place in their lives and affections. A mistake sometimes made by professionals is to take primary support roles on themselves. These roles are more appropriately carried out by the family and friends where the professional takes the role of being the facilitator or enabler in the situation. Such behaviour can make the family feel frustrated and pushed aside at a time when they most need to have something of value to offer. Obviously there are occasions when particular support may come more effectively from someone outside of the situation who has specific skills, but even then it should be seen as an enhancement of the support already in place and not as a replacement.

Clearly, identifying the resources a person already has may include considering aspects such as culture or faith, community support and involvement, as well as their own range of interests and facilities available for maintaining these. This can include existing group relationships such as the clergy or support from their own local religious groups.

Sensitivity and care is necessary when introducing a new support mechanism. If it is to work well, it first of all needs to win the acceptance of the person to whom it is offered and then to be further confirmed as the benefits are experienced and recognised by the individual and/or others in the immediate family circle.

SUPPORT FROM PROFESSIONALS

One vital resource underlying this continuing spiritual care for the patient and family is the caring professionals themselves. They provide a safety net which may give courage and confidence to continue when the going becomes difficult. The professionals have the capacity and ability to bring specific areas of discernment and expertise, and can have a very important role to play in expanding the ability of the patient and family to continue to respond to the changing situation.

SUPPORT GROUPS AS A RESOURCE

Support groups of one kind or another are an important resource of spiritual care for carers of all kinds, both professional and lay, and also for patients and their families. There are a number of different kinds of support groups, from the informal and *ad hoc* group ranging through to the formal and well-structured groups often led by professionals. It is essential to distinguish between the different types of groups which have very different purposes and serve different needs.

The informal group that comes together around a particular situation is able to act in a supportive way because the group is already in existence for another purpose. One example of this kind of group is the staff team that regularly meets together for ward reports or for team discussions and, where it is well run, staff may then feel able to share their difficulties and give appropriate support to one another.

There exists a range of more formalised groups which have different aims and objectives. There are those formed specifically for professional and personal debriefing after a particular incident or series of incidents, and in contrast regular groups which exist with very clear and focused aims and parameters. These may be groups where people can opt in or out as required, or commit themselves for a specified number of meetings. Examples of these groups are 'cancer support groups' or groups for sufferers of multiple sclerosis, cystic fibrosis, or loss of a baby (Thomas and Bryant, 1992). Sometimes these groups cater for patients and relatives together.

The value of such groups is variable and it is important to recognise groups do not work for everyone. In addition, timing can be important in terms of the right moment to introduce an individual in a specific situation. This is especially true for sufferers of particular diseases or for families after traumatic events in their lives. It is also important to monitor the progress of the group and to be prepared to adapt and change as the group changes.

Example

If you take bereavement support groups as an example, that the group exists may be the first line of support to someone experiencing trauma, and just the offer of an address or telephone number to contact for help may in itself be an important level of support. In the early stages or after the initial shock has abated and the deep pain of bereavement is being experienced, to meet with other sufferers may be therapeutic for some. To meet with people at different stages in that process can be helpful. To see and to speak with someone who is on the pathway through grief and who is beginning to rebuild their life may, in itself, be valuable and may bring a glimmer of hope to someone desperate with grief.

The group may also provide a safe environment for rediscovering how to relate to others in the community by meeting people who have experienced the isolation that can occur after bereavement. The group is a safe place to discover that conversations can take place without disintegration or devastation with the rediscovery of the belief that others can give help. Even in the depths of suffering there are people who will listen and respond, showing understanding and compassion. As the journey through the pain continues a balance of giving and receiving comes into play, as well as the ability to support others in pain within which a sense of value and purpose may be re-established.

Further along the journey, the balance may move more strongly into giving support and care to others and this may lead them into organisational roles. Others may enter into training to deepen their ability to respond to the needs of others.

This example is reflected in many other support groups, as those coming to terms with and accepting their own situation engage in support work with fellow sufferers. They may enter into activity such as fund-raising for their cause and, through such service, they find a new sense of purpose and value returning to their lives as their motivation for living is re-established.

THE VALUE OF SUPPORT GROUPS

It is generally agreed that support groups, whatever their form, bring certain benefits to most people. They can give a sense of security and anonymity as problems and achievements are shared (Tschudin, 1988). For some people comes the realisation that they are not alone and that others have come through a similar ordeal. Fears, feelings and reactions are shared bringing mutual support (Alexander, 1993). It cannot be assumed, however, that just getting together at regular intervals automatically ensures a therapeutic group as at times there can be a strong 'negative influence' – hence the need for some supervision from a leader or facilitator. It is known, however, that social support does reduce stress (Richman and Rosenfield, 1987).

So group members find certain common ground as they find other sufferers. Cancer sufferers, for example, begin to share and to discover how others cope with their difficulties, their problems encountered and their fears associated with that particular disease. Some help may be gained with very practical issues such as ways of carrying out certain functions, the right directions for finding help may be indicated. There may be opportunities to share the nature of their internal response to the disease in some depth, and to share concerns about the family and find out how they can be mutually helpful to each other.

There can of course be dangers when those who, because of their own experience, try to treat everyone's experiences as replicas of their own. This is where professional staff can be of help, particularly to the core members of the group. Many groups have a balance of self-help with an input from relevant professionals to maintain balance between the input of personal experience and the knowledge developed by study experience and professional practice.

There are groups where people can opt in or out and this is often likely to be the case for staff support groups, if organised on a permanent basis, where the membership may be different at almost every meeting. Individuals may attend as they need to or stop for a while and then return.

STAFF-SUPPORT GROUPS

Sometimes staff-support groups run for a specific purpose or length of time in response to a difficult situation, a period of change or pressure of work. Here staff may commit themselves for a specific period of time. This clearly has the advantage of being a stable group, which, if it gels, will enable deep discussion and exploration of the situation which has caused its existence.

In conjunction with debriefing after traumatic incidents, this can be helpful having a value in enabling staff to help each other to cope with difficult situations. Some groups are peer groups, which could be enabled to run more effectively by bringing in a facilitator as a member of the group. Other *ad hoc* groups have the advantage that they are not specifically set up within a contract – they come into being spontaneously and by nature they often tend to be peer groups. This enables staff to talk through and express feelings in a very unthreatening way, and to gain support from one another.

Support groups for staff are explored in more detail in Chapter 18, together with the criteria for good group leadership and for running a successful group. These ground rules are important and are applicable in most group situations.

It is important here to emphasise that not every person can be put into a group, and one-to-one support may well be the only acceptable route for some people.

Many groups set up to serve people with a specific disability or illness may include members from hospital and the community together, thus providing some continuity of care support and friendship in hospital and at home. Some of these are organised by voluntary associations or charities, and details of useful contacts are given in the appendix.

EXERCISE 34

Working with a member of your group, outline a short preparation course over a 6-week period for a group of volunteers in your department. How would you select volunteers for working in the field of spiritual care?

EXERCISE 35

Consider your own family group. Identify some of the resources available within your family. Share these with other members of your group and notice how much the resources become enriched by looking to friends and relationships, or within any community group.

QUESTION 1

What do you understand by a support group. Outline the different kinds of groups and describe their purposes. How would you evaluate their usefulness?

Key points

- One of the most valuable resources for spiritual care is the patient's own family.
- Volunteers are an excellent resource if selected and prepared for the purpose with care.
- It is important to identify the patient's need and resources which may be enhanced by skilled professional help and family support.
- Support groups are a valuable resource for patients, families and staff, and may exist in a variety of forms.

CHAPTER 18

Caring for the carers – staff have needs too

Where's your boat?
'I ought to say' said Pooh –
'That it isn't just an ordinary sort of boat,
Sometimes it's a boat and sometimes it's more of an accident
It all depends' –
'Depends on what?'
'On whether I'm on the top of it or underneath it!'

A A Milne – *Winnie the Pooh*

The aim of good patient care lies at the heart of our consideration of spiritual care, and the quality of patient care is highly dependent on the quality of care the staff receive. To give good quality care requires a special kind of confidence and self-esteem. Staff need to feel valued and respected and it has to be recognised that they too are as vulnerable as any other individual to life's pressures and traumas.

There has been a long tradition among health-care staff that they must remain competent and in control of all events and that they must always appear to be coping with every situation all the time. Failure to cope or showing emotion is often seen as a sign of weakness, when in fact it is often a sign of real sensitivity and vulnerability and ability to feel a concern about those in their care. There is also a tendency to see ourselves as either the carers or the cared for rather than recognising that we all have similar human needs (Stoter, 1991). There is evidence that good staff morale improves the quality of patient care and speeds up recovery (Revans,1962; Hingley, 1991). It is difficult to give a high standard of patient care, however, if we neglect ourselves and do not feel valued.

This Chapter draws heavily on what has already been explored earlier in the text, particularly with reference to personal growth and development. Therefore, it helps to read the Chapter as a synthesis of issues particularly relevant to staff support and set in that context.

WHAT IS STAFF SUPPORT?

Staff support is a means of helping those who care for others to be fully effective in their service. So often lip service is paid to prevention, but we have become geared to a disease-orientated medical service which waits for problems to develop and then responds with the appropriate treatment. In the case of support to staff, the services are brought in or put in place when the problems come, which means sadly they often come too little and too late. The remedies can be built into the structure as part of the fabric, however, before the crisis arises.

So often staff support is only recognised under the name of a counselling or occupational health service when in fact there are many different ways in which it exists through other networks which are already in place in the organisation. There are good one-to-one relationships or formal or informal group settings which can be used if staff are encouraged to share their feelings of helplessness and frustration in a forum which is not threatening.

Where a good counselling service exists it needs the back-up of good staff support practices all the time if it is not to be used just to pick up the casualties at the end of the line. 'Staff support involves a healthy working environment and a caring culture as an integral part of every institutional setting. It ensures that a wide range of support mechanisms is available and fosters a management structure in which individuals are valued.' (NASS, 1992).

WHY IS STAFF SUPPORT NECESSARY?

There is ample evidence to show that the effects of stress can be very costly both in human terms to the individual, and to the employer in resource terms (NASS, 1992). We all need a certain amount of stress to function normally and certainly stress can be creative if channelled into satisfying activities. However, when stress is allowed to build up unchecked, the balance is disturbed, the point of creativity is passed and there is a negative response which can have all kinds of undesirable effects. These effects can lead to a range of symptoms for individuals such as irritability, insomnia, difficulties in concentrating or in decision-making or ultimately burn-out or stress-related illnesses (Cooper, 1988).

These effects have all been documented in many studies together with the wider effects such as being absent from work and poor work performance (Owen, 1993). What is less well reported, is the demoralising effects on team work as the downward spiral has a cumulative effect within a group, ultimately adversely, affecting group performance. The downward spiral leads to a loss of teamwork and a loss of individual self-esteem. This is often exemplified by poor eating habits, loss of normal sleep patterns, tiredness, apathy and a loss of social activity, all of which may feed into deteriorating relationships at home.

> *Those who listen day after day – in exposing themselves to*
> *another's pain are part of the healing process ...*

*Pain is part of the human condition and sharing that pain
is a deeply human task.*

Sheila Cassidy – *Good Friday People*

The preceding Chapters of this book have shown clearlythat those who care enough to come alongside and seek to journey with those who suffer life's painful experiences are constantly exposed to high levels of distress and to disturbing situations (Rushton, 1992). A carer who is sensitive to the pain of others is inevitably vulnerable to personal pain and at risk to high stress levels. This exposure can have a cumulative effect over a period of time or, alternatively, a sudden traumatic incident or a large-scale major disaster, can lead to post-traumatic stress disorder with long-term implications for staff affected. The more sensitive and caring a person is, the more vulnerable they are to such pressures. That is not to suggest that such people should not join the caring professions – rather the reverse as they often provide the more desirable qualities for good standards of care. It does underline the need for adequate preventive and support measures to be in place, however, and to be available to everyone at all times (Johnson, 1992).

PROVIDING SUPPORT FOR PROFESSIONAL CARERS

The provision of good staff support is an essential preventive measure for maintaining a happy and healthy workforce, but it also has a potential for promoting a high quality service for the patients and families in their care. Staff who understand and recognise all forms of human need (here we are particularly concerned with spiritual care) and who are aware of and respect their own personal and spiritual needs in a responsible manner, are much more likely to recognise and meet the needs of those in their care.

Staff support can be considered on three levels, each one contributing to the creation and maintenance of the caring culture:
• The personal level.
• The group or team level.
• The organisational level.

Many would consider that staff support is primarily a management responsibility, but this approach alone can lead to feelings of helplessness and negativity for the staff who feel powerless to effect change themselves. Stress management, if approached in all three ways simultaneously, helps to redress feelings of powerlessness and it channels energies creatively and establishes the attitude that something can be done (Stoter, 1991; Rushton, 1992).

The personal or individual approach

We need to begin with ourselves. To those who have grown up in the tradition of putting others first, this may be difficult to accept at first, but a little thought will make it clear that an overstressed and burnt-out carer is not able to provide the most efficient and caring service. Staff who take responsibility for themselves will help others to feel they are valued and respected and are much more likely to create a good working environment and to generate good team communications and provide quality care.

We need to start responsibly by considering our health, lifestyle and use of rest and recreation. The person who is so disorganised that they rarely get off duty on time or take adequate holidays is not going to be a very interesting or communicative person when meeting individuals from the outside world. In addition, they will not have much idea of what is going on in the wider world. Adequate rest or time to recuperate personal resources is essential and not a luxury. Holidays and days off are important, but so too are smaller breaks. It is also important to know when to take a few minutes out to have a cup of tea or to relax and take stock of the next course of action if one is going into a situation that needs concentrated listening and the sharing of difficult circumstances and responses.

It is important to recognise that spiritual care can be very demanding and draining and we need to recognise this in our colleagues and to be aware of when they need relief for a period, or to step aside for a moment's support themselves. This applies to all levels of staff, and not least to the managers. These are all very basic and ordinary things which are often overlooked and considered to be unimportant in professional care, but they can make a real difference.

Then there is the personal professional development side to consider. We all need to take seriously opportunities for keeping up to date professionally and also for regular re-appraisal of our own personal response to the pain and suffering we share with others. This means looking at our own personal methods of coping with stressful situations and defusing the build up of stress. It involves understanding many of the issues discussed in Chapters 2 and 3 of this book. It requires a degree of self-awareness and acceptance of oneself and opportunities to apply knowledge gained in the classroom to the realities of the ward or department, and a chance to assess our performance afterwards. Self-knowledge is a fundamental basis for understanding others.

All of this demands constant re-appraisal and vigilance and also a readiness to seek experienced help if we feel overwhelmed, out of our depth, or unable to cope at times. Also such an approach to self-awareness and personal growth can best take place in a culture which accepts and caters for such responsible behaviour. This leads us to look next at the overall organisational and management aspects of support.

Support from the organisational perspective

It makes sense to consider this element next as much of what follows in this context may also be relevant in the group situation and in the workplace. It is widely considered (and indeed this approach appears to have the support of the Department of Health) that support is a management responsibility. It is a fact, however, that this is not borne out in practice – studies show that only one in ten health authorities have a recognised staff-support policy (NASS, 1993; Cooper, 1993). In ideal circumstances there should be budget provision for this aspect of care but, in the current climate, this receives a low priority and even where it exists, it does not follow that resources for support are adequate. Such provision does not remove the responsibility of management from other aspects of care for staff.

Managers have a responsibility to establish and maintain a general ethos for the care of staff. This includes creating a recognition of the effects of stress and owning a responsibility to ensure that support of staff is both accepted and available. Expressing a need for support is not an admission of weakness, but rather an important acknowledgement that caring professionals should not be 'loners' but part of a team. Staff need to know that they can ask for help and where to turn for further help. Involving staff in the decision-making processes and creating good communication channels are part of this approach, so that they feel respected and valued as part of the team and able to use their skills effectively. This also enables staff to take a pride in the service provided.

Many other areas also need attention; for example, good selection procedures which ensure as far as possible that the right person has the right job and so contributes to building up job satisfaction. This needs to be followed by proper training and preparation for the job in hand, and by good in-service training so that they feel confident and have opportunities to extend and develop their skills. All this needs to be backed up by good environmental working conditions and by a strong occupational health service, ideally supported by a counselling service. It is quite probable that many of these resources for support already exist in many places, but they are not always coordinated or widely known and so they need to be identified, recognised and valued by management. It sometimes falls to the role of the occupational health or chaplaincy departments to develop this role where there is no overall management policy. It can clearly be seen from this discussion that there is a need for a coordinating role if this type of care is to be available to each individual at their point of need.

Group or team support

Group or team support in the work place is perhaps the most widely established and appreciated form of staff care available. This, when well understood and used, can be effective both in dealing with the effects of particularly traumatic situations immediately and also in resolving issues of a less dramatic nature, which, if ignored, can fester and cause disharmony. The previous Chapter has already given an introduction to the general aspects of support groups and their value and this will be continued here with special reference to staff needs.

Support groups for staff can vary in the way they function and in their purpose, according to need. The range is wide including :
- The informal or ad-hoc group, which forms spontaneously or already exists, for example, ward report team/meeting.
- A group formed for a short period to meet a specific crisis.
- A self-awareness training group offering a specific series of meetings.
- A self-development or assertiveness training group, to assist in developing coping mechanisms.
- A problem solving or action learning group.
- A facilitator-led group, which can allow in-depth work.
- Groups offering relaxation or other special techniques for stress relief.

Some of these groups obviously need an expert leader or facilitator, so choice of approach will depend much on the local resources available and the needs to be met.

EXERCISE 36
Is staff support necessary for the provision of quality spiritual care? Explore this situation in your group and identify the nature and sources of staff support in your particular work place.

EXERCISE 37
Identify the personal support system you have in your own life and consider:
• Whether you feel it is adequate for your personal needs.
• How it has helped you to grow and develop as a person.
Identify any areas of personal need you have where you would like more support.

Support groups offer staff the opportunity to have their own spiritual and emotional needs recognised and acknowledged in turn, and to receive care and understanding through moments of doubt and personal pain. Such opportunities are useful in helping each of them to understand and accept their own humanity, and so to be better equipped to share and accept the frailties of others. In addition, it can make them more confident in their approach to spiritual care.

Training groups are a valuable resource for support as they may be available through educational channels and therefore more readily accepted as part of professional in-service training. Again, such developmental training enables staff to offer a more understanding level of care to others through personal enlightenment. Their skills can then be extended to others and there are opportunities for further learning experiences, if the training is enhanced by good, on the spot, back-up support in the work place.

CRITERIA FOR SUCCESSFUL GROUP WORK

Ideally, every formal support group should have a leader or facilitator, with appropriate skills. There are situations where this is not possible, however, and peer-group support is the best option open. In any case, there are certain basic criteria which are essential for success. It is advisable to have a time set aside for meetings and members need to be aware of the purpose of the group and to agree on the ground rules for procedure. The need for trust and assurance of confidentiality is basic to all group work and participants need to be fully agreed on this point (Bond, 1990).

Where more in-depth work is anticipated, a professionally trained leader is desirable. The style of leadership can affect the success of the group, and different styles of leadership suit different purposes. Flexibility, sensitivity and awareness of needs are essential for the facilitation process (Alexander, 1993). Readers seeking more practical information on this issue would find guidance in one of the NASS series pamphlets which gives step-by-step guidance (NASS, 1993).

One hazard facing groups working without skilled leadership is the danger of becoming a 'whinge' group, which can be negative and contribute to a downward spiral. It is very easy to slip into the 'poor me' syndrome, and for collusion to take place which reinforces the problems and feelings of helplessness. There is also a tendency to identify a problem, give it a name and then distance oneself from it by thinking that is has been dealt with, which has the effect of freezing the issue. A skilled leader can help the members to explore the deeper concerns and their own responses to them, facing the painful aspects and coming to terms with reality. A successful group situation allows members to resolve these issues by taking appropriate steps and responses. This has a therapeutic effect for the individuals and also helps them to care for the organisation at large, creating a culture of success, which, in itself, is part of the healing process and leads individuals further on their quest for self-development and spiritual growth.

There is considerable evidence to show that staff support groups play an important part in staff development and growth, and in alleviating stress. They are particularly beneficial where constant debriefing is required or in situations like hospice work, or intensive care units where the pressures run high (Farrell, 1992; Richman *et al.*, 1987; Spinks *et al.*, 1990). Good support groups help to create good teamwork.

> *Many people just do not know themselves, because they proudly believe they can give birth to themselves. The fact is that none of us can reveal ourselves to ourselves, unless we first reveal ourselves to another, who listens to us with love.*
>
> Michel Quoist – *The Breath of Love*

QUESTION 1

Why is staff support so important for carers? Discuss, giving evidence from any literature you have read.

QUESTION 2

How would you recognise the symptoms of an inbalance of stress in yourself and your colleagues and what can be done:
(a) To prevent this happening?
(b) To deal with it when recognised?

QUESTION 3

Outline a system of staff-support suitable for your workplace. Describe how you would go about developing this. How would you decide which colleagues to work with?

QUESTION 4

What are the ground rules essential to establish a good staff support group? Describe the different kinds of group you are familiar with.

Key points

- Traditions in health care reinforce attitudes that staff should be able to cope.
- Staff who care are sensitive and so vulnerable, and the effects of stress can be costly, both to the individual and the employer.
- Provision of staff support can be considered in three areas: the individual, the group and the organisation.
- Managers need support as well as holding a responsibility to provide it.
- Support groups are valuable if well organised with agreed ground rules.
- Good group support enhances good teamwork and facilitates provision of good care.

Section VI

Wholeness and healing in spiritual care

We shall not cease from exploration
And the end of all our exploring
Will be to arrive where we started
And know the place for the first time.

TS Eliot

INTRODUCTION

This exploration into spiritual care started with identifying differences between spiritual and religious need and care, looking at some basic definitions fundamental to understanding the notion of people journeying together through suffering and painful experiences. Each aspect of the process was then explored in more detail looking at the various people involved and their needs, skills and roles. Their responses to pain and recovery were looked at, as well as some specific areas of need and the resources available to both carers and patients.

It has been apparent throughout the discussion that many factors are interrelated in each aspect of the process of spiritual care. Each individual patient, relative and carer involved brings a range of different needs to the process such as resources, experience and skills, which overlap making each relationship and situation unique.

Our exploration of this process, which has been identified as 'spiritual care', would not be complete, however, without some synthesis of these different facets and an attempt to identify the unifying or common factor in the process. This final Chapter will bring our exploration in full circle through a holistic approach to spiritual care, which is becoming a very prominent perspective in current thinking.

CHAPTER 19

Bringing it all together – the healing relationship

The concept of wholeness relates to a process going on within a person, enabling a particular response to the situation encountered on the spiritual journey to take place. There is sometimes confusion in understanding the difference between healing and cure, as is often evident in media presentations and in the eyes of the general public. This confusion is also apparent in literature and in journal articles, as many writers assume there is a common acceptance of the language used and do not always clarify their own perspective. There is often a common assumption that cure is the only acceptable outcome where illness or disease is concerned. This has been reinforced during recent years by professionals, many of whom regard cure as the major criterion for judgment of successful treatment, having an expectation that cure is the only completely successful outcome.

It is also helpful to understand the differences between illness and disease, and Downe and Telfer (1980) have a full discussion on this in relation to values and beliefs. They point out that there is a 'built in reference to some normal condition of the human body by reference to which these things are aberrations'.

Disease is usually a more technical notion than illness and generally there is a recognisable cause. There is also a difference between being ill and feeling ill.

CURE AND HEALING

Cure is concerned with the eradication of disease and is a general expectation of most people today when they become ill. It carries the implication of the removal of symptoms or the end of a specific disease process through some kind of medical or mechanical intervention (McGlone, 1991).

Healing has a wider connotation, however, being concerned with whatever is happening within the person who is in the process of being cured, or who is beginning the journey of coming to terms with deteriorating health or with the prospect of death.

Healing is about journeying towards wholeness of mind, body and spirit as an entirety. It is about people coming to peace with themselves, even if the person does not like what is happening. It embraces the patient coming to peace within him- or herself and the family, and also with the relationship with the carers. It is a process of getting in touch with whatever is impeding progress towards wholeness; it is an integration of receiving and responding to care which is creative. Each person responds within themselves according to their own capacity for coping, from where they have reached on their journey. The depth and quality of communication within the various relationships involved is of the utmost importance, and those who facilitate healing and wholeness focus more on the person than on the disease.

It is possible to experience deep levels of healing and wholeness without being cured and also to be cured of disease, but to have achieved little or nothing in relationship to the process of healing and wholeness.

As McGlone points out (1991), looking at the range of topics related to this subject and the variety of resources available, we can easily be misled by assuming we are all talking about the same thing. In fact, meanings can vary enormously according to the writer's perspective.

As we have seen throughout this text, there is a range of possible approaches towards healing and cure and, while one approach is appropriate for a particular individual or disease, there may be many alternatives to select from to meet the needs and preferences of different individuals. Where practicable, these should be respected and implemented. This is where the central component of an integrated and inclusive approach to spiritual care is essential and requires the highest levels of teamwork.

Sometimes, it appears to be a sadness that people reach the highest levels of integration and wholeness at the end of their lives, facilitated by the process of coming to terms with what is, arguably, the greatest challenge of life – dying. This process needs to be reassessed and seen as a criteria for judging success. Success is giving a high level of care which has enabled healing and wholeness to take place where cure has been impossible. At the core of this process is love, the right sort of love of self, which allows a valuing of self in receiving what is necessary and right and responding openly, which is creative for self, family and staff. Openness, honesty and acceptance are important words and concepts, which when practised by patient, family and staff, create an environment which encourages self-esteem for all involved and thus an environment conducive to growth.

THE CORE OF SPIRITUAL CARE – EASING DIS-EASE

The synthesis of this theme would be incomplete without reference to a concept referred to many times throughout this exploration: the concept of 'partnership' based on a relationship between carer and patient, whether the carer is a professional, family member or friend. This relationship is essential for the sharing of care, trust and love, and is all part of the whole 'framework' which facilitates the process of offering spiritual care. This concept of 'partnership' means different things to different people and, while many acknowledge the importance of it, it is often imperfectly understood and interpreted and few authors actually address the theme (Bayntun-Lees, 1992). What is often overlooked is that everyone involved in such a partnership in caring can share in a rich growing experience with mutual personal enhancement (Peplau, 1988), especially where the relationship is based on equality and mutual commitment with good communication.

Love means a willingness to participate in the being of the other at the cost of suffering, and with the expectation of mutual enrichment, criticism and growth. (D Day Williams, 1968.)

The central core or essence of spiritual care, when properly delivered, quite clearly sets the patient at the heart of the picture surrounded by family and friends who, in turn, are supported by professionals. The ideal of spiritual care enables the individual patient to identify and experience a value within himself, and to value and respond to care given by family and friends releasing them to express love and care in return.

It is clearly essential for professionals to respond to needs as identified and, in partnership with family and friends, to strive to bring 'ease from dis-ease'. Spiritual care is thus that integrating power or force in total patient care which signals the overwhelming need to recognise the person who is suffering and, by extension, to recognise the suffering in family, among friends and indeed for the professionals involved as well.

This speaks of a deep partnership built on trust, understanding and deep respect for the individual and, above all, a partnership fuelled with love. 'Love' is a much abused and misunderstood word frequently devalued but in its widest sense, it is the only word which most clearly describes the desire to give or to have the very best interests of the other person at heart. At its best, it is a gift which defies description, but can be recognised and valued by its effects.

Vanstone says :

> Where love is authentic, the lover gives to the object of his
> love a certain power over himself – a power which would not
> otherwise be there.

When this level of care is given and received, it is often the case that the individual achieves the highest level of integration in their lives and a new wholeness of personality. This comes at a time when they are least able to 'do', but are able to share that wholeness in a manner which enables the legacy left behind with the family to be a good and positive one. For those with a particular faith, this may also embrace that unity with God in whatever way He is known or understood in their experience.

As the expression of valuing the individual comes at a time when they are unable to remain actively involved in doing things, by extension they frequently believe their value to others has been destroyed. To discover that sense of being valued at such a time and to know they are valued by family, friends and professionals, may touch very deep chords and bring about a healing of the person. Despite the fact that their body may be deteriorating and strength fading, this can bring a new integration and wholeness of personality which can reveal inner strengths hitherto undiscovered.

Love is perhaps one of the greatest easing forces in disease, bringing acceptance and understanding showing value by touch, word or eye contact or just simply by being there.

MAKING IT WORK IN REALITY

All this is a daunting task for any one individual who tries to go it alone, but as we have seen throughout this book, each one of us is part of a team working through relationships with each other, with the family and with the patient. Working together and sharing skills, personal expertise and sensitivity enhances the whole process which becomes greater and stronger than the 'sum of each individual contribution'.

As Michel Quoist says in *The Breath of Love*:

If each note of music were to say: one note doesnnot make a symphony
there would be no symphony
If each one of us were to say: one act of love cannot save mankind
there would never be justice and peace on earth–
The symphony needs each note
The book needs each word
The house needs each brick
The ocean needs each drop of water
The harvest needs each grain of wheat
The whole of humanity needs you as and where you are
You are unique,
No one can take your place –
Begin now, – why are you waiting?

Key points

- This final Chapter represents a synthesis of the exploration throughout the book.
- The concepts of wholeness, healing and cure are re-examined.
- The core of spiritual care is identified as love.
- Love is one of the greatest forces in easing disease.

APPENDIX – USEFUL ADDRESSES AND RESOURCES

Useful sources of information

This list of resources includes some useful addresses for reference in specific situations referred to in the text. It does not attempt to offer an exhaustive list of services, as those can usually be obtained through local trusts, health authorities or local libraries. Those listed are mostly specialist organisations offering support and information rather than financial help. Many have free information leaflets on receipt of a SAE.

An excellent small guide worth purchasing separately is the *BBC Family Directory*, listing over 150 organisations providing help and information to families. At £1 per copy it is good value. Available from:
Customer Services
Health Education Authority
Hamilton House
Mabledon Place
London WC1H 9TX
Tel: 071 413 1946
(or through any bookshop)

Other particularly useful addresses are:

Breast Care and Mastectomy Association of Great Britain (BCMA)
26a Harrison Street
Kings Cross
London WC1H 8JG
Tel: 071 837 0908
A free service of practical advice, information and support to women concerned about breast cancer. Volunteers who have had breast cancer themselves assist the staff in providing emotional support, nationwide.

British Association for Counselling
37a Sheep Street
Rugby
Warks CV21 3BX
Tel: 0788 78328/9
BAC members are individuals and organisations concerned with counselling in a variety of settings. The Information Office publishes directories listing accredited counsellors.

British Colostomy Association
38–39 Eccleston
Square
London SW1V 1PB
Tel: 071 828 5175
An information and advisory service giving comfort, reassurance and encouragement to patients to return to their previous active lifestyle. Emotional support is given on a personal and confidential basis by helpers who have long experience of living with a colostomy.

Cancer Aftercare and Rehabilitation Society (CARE)
21 Zetland Road
Redland
Bristol BS6 7AH
Tel: 0272 427419
This is an organisation of cancer patients formed into self-help groups who offer advice and support.

Cancerlink
17 Britannia Street
London WC1X 9JN
Tel: 071 833 2451
The group provides emotional support and information in response to telephone and letter enquiries on all aspects of cancer, from people with cancer to families, friends and professionals working with them. There is resource to over 300 cancer support and self-help groups throughout Britain, and the organisation helps people who set up new groups.

Cancer Relief MacMillan Fund
Anchor House
15/19 Britten Street
London SW3 3TZ
Tel: 071 351 7811

The MacMillan fund supports and develops services to provide skilled care for people with cancer and their families. The organisation provides MacMillan nurses, MacMillan units for in-patient and day care and financial help through grants.

Child Bereavment Trust
1 Millside
Riverdale
Bourne End
Bucks SL8 SEB

Provides support and counselling for bereaved families. Supplies videos, helpful literature and training for carers.

CRITECH – Crisis Counselling, Training, Education, Support, Information Service
Accident and Emergency
Leeds General Infirmary
Leeds LS1 3EX
Tel: 0532 432799

CRITECH offers training, debriefing and an information service for those working with sudden death and other life crises.

Foundation for the Study of Infant Death
(Cot Death Research and Support Associations)
5th Floor, 4 Grosvenor Place
London SW1 7HD
Tel: 071 235 172

Advice and counselling is provided for newly bereaved parents. The Foundation sponsors research and produces useful leaflets.

Gay Switchboard
BM Switchboard
London WC1N 3XX
Tel: 071 349 0839

Twenty-four hour information and help service for lesbians and gay men. This service will also refer those recently bereaved to their bereavement project.

Jewish Bereavement Counselling Service
14 Chalgrove Gardens
London NW3 3PN
Tel: 071 349 0839

This group sends trained volunteer counsellors to bereaved people. It operates in Greater London, but can refer to other projects and individuals elsewhere.

Hospice Information Service
St Christopher's Hospice
51–59 Lawrie Park Road
Sydenham
London SE26 6DZ
Tel: 081 778 9252

The Hospice Information Service publishes a directory of hospice services which provides details of hospices, home care teams and hospital support teams in the UK and the Republic of Ireland.

Institute for Complementary Medicine
21 Portland Place
London W1N 3AF

This institute can supply names of reliable practitioners of complementary medicine such as homeopathy, relaxation techniques and osteopathy. It also has contact with other support groups. Send a SAE for information, stating your area of interest.

Institute of Family Therapy
43 New Cavendish Street,
London W1M 7RG
Tel: 071 935 1651

The Institute's Elizabeth Raven Memorial Fund offers free counselling to recently bereaved families or those with seriously ill members of family. It works with the whole family.

Let's Face It
Christine Piff
10 Wood End
Crowthorne
Berks RG11 6DQ
Tel: 0344 774405

A contact point for people of any age coping with facial disfigurement. The group provides a link for people with similar experiences by telephone and letter contact, meetings for self-help or by social contact.

The Lisa Sainsbury Foundation
8–10 Crown Hill
Croydon
Surrey
Tel: 081 686 8808

This Foundation offers information and training support to those caring for the dying and the bereaved. Videos, literature and trainers can be made available to organisations.

Marie Curie Cancer Care
28 Belgrave Street
London SW1X 8QG
Tel: 071 235 3325

Nursing care is available in 11 Marie Curie homes throughout the UK. Admission details are obtained through the individual matrons. Day and night nursing can be provided in the patient's home through the Community Nursing Service.

National Association for Staff Support (NASS)
9 Caradon Close
Woking
Surrey GU21 3DU
Tel: 0483 771599

NASS is an association of professionals with a common interest in coordinating and developing staff support resources for all health-care staff. It produces its own literature, quarterly newsletter and organises conferences and workshops.

National Association for Widows (NAW)
c/o Stafford and District Voluntary Service Centre
Chell Road
Stafford ST16 2QA
Tel: 0785 45465

Advice, support and friendship is available to widows. This is a pressure group fighting against financial anomalies that widows have to face.

Stillbirth and Neonatal Death Society (SANDS)
Argyle House
29–31 Euston Road
London NW1 2SD
Tel: 071 833 2851

SANDS offers advice and long-term support via local groups to newly bereaved parents of stillbirths and/or of babies who die in their first month of life.

The Sue Ryder Foundation
Cavendish, Sudbury
Suffolk CO10 8AY
Tel: 0787 280252

Six Sue Ryder Homes in England specialise in cancer care. Visiting nurses care for patients in their own homes. Advice and bereavement counselling are provided.

Support After Termination of Abnormality (SATFA)
22 Upper Woburn Place,
London WC1H 0EP

This is a support group run by women and couples who have experienced a termination of pregnancy because of abnormality.

Tak Tent
Cancer Support Organisation
G Block, Western Infirmary,
Glasgow G11 6NT
Tel: 041 332 3639

This group gives emotional support, counselling and information on aspects of cancer. It has support groups throughout Scotland and a one-to-one counselling service at the centre by appointment.

Other loss and bereavement resources include:
For the junior stage:
Lorentzen K, 1982: *Lanky Longlegs*. Dent, London.
Stiles N, 1984: *I'll Miss You, Mr Hooper*. Random House, London.
White EB, 1969: *Charlotte's Web*. Puffin, London.
For secondary stage:
Branfield J, 1981: *Fox in Winter*. Armada/Collins, Glasgow.
Hoy L, 1983: *Your Friend Rebecca*. Beaver/Arrow, London.
Hunter M, 1975: *A Sound of Chariots*. Armada/Collins, Glasgow.
Lowry L, 1980: *A Summer to Die*. Granada, London.
Williams JG and Ross J, 1983: *When People Die*. Macdonald, London.
Machin L, 1990: *Looking at Loss: A Bereavement Counselling Pack*. Longman, Harlow.

FURTHER READING

SECTION I

Burkhart MA *et al.* (1994) Reawakening the Spirit in Clinical Practice. Journal of Holistic Nursing Vol 12 No 1: 9–27.
Campbell A (1984) A Moderated Love. SPCK, London.

SECTION II

Axline V (1981) DIBS – In Search of Self. Hamondsworth Pelican, London.
Bowlby B (1968 & 1980) Attachment & Loss Vols I–III.
Connington B (1966) The Therapeutic Touch. Prentice Hall Press, New York.
Kreiger D (1979) The Therapeutic Touch. Prentice Hall Press, New York.
Leibowitz J *et al.* (1990) The Alexander Technique. Souvenir Press, London.
Rogers C (1967) On Becoming a Person. Constable, London.
Rutter M (1981) Maternal Deprivation Reassessed. Penguin, London.
Scott Peck M (1993) Further Along the Road Less Travelled.

SECTION III

Cook B (1988) Loss and Bereavement. Lisa Sainsbury Foundation.
Cox C (1983) Sociology (Chapters 8 & 13). Butterworth, Sevenoaks, Kent.
Kubler-Ross E (1969) On Death & Dying. Macmillan, New York.
Lewis CS (1961) A Grief Observed. Faber & Faber, London.
Norman L (1988) The Reflexology Handbook. Bath Press.
Penson J (1991) Complimentary Therapies in Palliative Care for People with Cancer. Arnold, London.
Rankin-Box D (1988) Complementary Health Therapies: A Guide for Nursing and the Caring Professions. Croom Helm, London.
Raphael B (1985) The Anatomy of Bereavement: A Handbook for the Caring Professions. Hutchinson, London.
Speck P (1978) Loss and Grief in Medicine. Balliere Tindall, London.

SECTION IV

Campbell AV (1975) Moral Dilemmas in Medicine.
Downe S & Telfer E (1980) Caring & Curing: A Philosophy of Medicine & Social Work. Methuen, London.
Fromer MJ (1981) Ethical Issues in Healthcare. CV Mosby, St Louis.
Green J (1989 & 1991) Death with Dignity Vols I & II. A Nursing Times publication.
McGilloway O & Myco F (1985) Nursing & Spiritual Care. Harper & Row, London.
Neuberger J (1987) Caring for Dying People of Different Faiths. Sainsbury Series, Austen Cornish, London.
Penson J & Fisher R (1991) Palliative Care for People with Cancer. Arnold, London.
Rumbold G (1986) Ethics in Nursing Practice. Balliere Tindall, London.
Sampson C (1982) The Neglected Ethic: Cultural and Religious Factors in the Care of Patients. McGraw Hill, London.
Tschudin V (1992) Ethics in Nursing: The Caring Relationship. Butterworth & Heinemann.

SECTION V

Bond M (1990) Setting up a Support Group. NASS Occasional Paper No 3.
Cox C (1983) Sociology: An Introduction for Nurses, Midwives and Health Visitors (Parts I & IV). Butterworth.
Krech *et al.* (1962) The Individual in Society. McGraw Hill. (See Chapter 14 for an introduction to role theory.)
NASS (1992) A Charter for Staff Support. NASS, London.
Nichols K & Jenkinson J (1991) Leading a Staff Support Group.
A Working Party Report (1991) Mud & Stars. A Sobell House publication, Oxford.

Tschudin V (1988) Staff Support in Nursing the Patient with Cancer. Prentice Hall, Hemel Hempstead.

Vachon MLS (1988) Battle Fatigue in Hospice/Palliative Care. In Gilmore A & Gilmore S (Eds) A Softer Death. Plenum, New York.

(NB The National Association for Staff Support has a series of useful publications on this subject – see Appendix)

SECTION VI

Downe S & Telfer E (1980) A Philosophy of Medicine and Social Work. Methuen, London.

Levin JS (1994) Religion & Health: Is there an Association? Is it Valid? Is it Causal? Social Science & Medicine Vol 38 No 11: 1475–1482.

REFERENCES

Aldridge D (1991) Spirituality, healing and medicine. British Journal of General Practice **41**: 425–427.

Alexander DA (1993) Staff support groups: do they support and are they even groups? Palliative Medicine Vol 5: 127–132.

Allen C (1991) The inner light. Nursing Standard Vol 5, No 20: 52–53.

Baytun-Lees D, 1992: Reviewing the nurse–patient partnership. Nursing Standard Vol No 6, 42: 36–39.

Benjamin M (1986) Ethics in Nursing. OUP, Oxford, 2nd Edition.

Curtis J, Bloor MJ, Horobin GW (1975) Conflict and Resolution in Doctor/Patient Interactions. In Cox C, Mead A (Eds) A Sociology of Medical Practice OP Cit271.

Bernstein B (1960) Language & Social Class. British Journal Sociology 15, London.

Bond M (1990) Setting up a Support Group Occasional Paper No 3 NASS.

Bowers C (1990) Spiritual Dimension of the Rehabilitation Journey. Rehabilitation Nursing Vol 12 No 2.

Bowlby J (1953) Child Care and the Growth of Love. Pelican, London.

Bowlby J (1969) Attachment & Loss (Vol 1). Basic Books, New York.

Bowlby J (1977) Attachment & Loss (Vol 2). Basic Books, New York.

Bowlby J (1980) Attachment & Loss (Vol 3). Basic Books, New York.

Bradshaw WJ (1972) The Concept of Social Need, New Society 30: 640–643.

Brothers J (1971) Religious Institutions. Longman, Harlow.

Burgess K (1992) Supporting Bereaved Relatives in A&E. Nursing Standard Vol 6 No 19: 36–39.

Burkhardt MA *et al.* (1985) Dealing with Spiritual Concerns of Clients in the Community. Journal of Community Health Nursing Vol 2 No 4: 191–198.

Burkhardt MA *et al.* (1994) Reawakening spirit in clinical practice. Journal Holistic Nursing Vol 12 No 1: 9–21.

Burnard P (1988) The Spiritual Needs of Atheists and Agnostics. Professional Nurse December 1988: 130 and 132.

Burnard P (1990) Learning to Care for the Spirit. Nursing Standard Vol 4 No 18.

Byrne C (1992) Research Methods in Complementary Therapies. Nursing Standard Vol 6 No 52.

Campbell A (1975) Moral Dilemmas in Medicine. Churchill Livingstone, Edinburgh. Campbell A (1984) A Moderated Love – A Theology of Professional Care. SPCK, London.

Carson V (1980) Meeting the spiritual needs of hospitalised psychiatric patients. Perspect Psychiatric Care Vol 18 No1: 17–20.

Chesterfield (1992) Communicating with Dying Children. Nursing Standard Vol 6 No 20.

Clifford M (1987) Facilitating Spiritual Care in the Rehabilitation Setting. Rehabilitation Nursing Vol 12 No 6: 331–332.

Cook B, Phillips S (1988) Loss and Bereavement. Lisa Sainsbury Foundation Series. Austen Cornish, London.

Cox CJ, Mead AJ (Eds) (1975 A Sociology of Medical Practice. Collier–MacMillan, London.

Cox C (1983) Sociology (Chapters 8 & 13). Butterworths, Sevenoaks, Kent.

Davis J (1993) Ethical & Legal Issues in Suicide. Br Journal of Nursing Vol 2 No 15: 777–780.

Denton P *et al.* (1992) Make your Voice Heard. Nursing Standard Vol 6 No 50.

Dickleman N (1992) When Words Fail (The Importance of Touch). Nursing Times Vol 88 No 49: 41.

Dimmond B (1993) Who Deserves Care? Editorial British Journal of Nursing. Vol 2 No 15: 743.

Douglas I, Ellis S (1991) Reflexology. Element Books, London.

Downie S, Telfer E (1980) Caring and Curing. A Philosophy of Medicine and Social Work. Methuen, London.

Doyle D (1992) Have we looked beyond the physical and psychosocial? Journal of Pain & Symptom Management Vol 7 No 5.

Dugan DO (1987) Death & dying. Journal of Psychiatric Nursing Vol 25 No 7.

Elkin F (1960) The Child & Society (Chapters 2 & 3). Raiden Hume, N Yorks.

Ellis P *et al.* (1992) A Child's right to die – who should decide? British Journal of Nursing Vol 1 No 8: 404–407.

Ellison G (1992) A Private disaster. Nursing Times Vol 88 No 52.

Farrell M (1992) A process of mutual support: establishing a support network for nurses caring for dying patients. Professional Nurse, October 1992: 10–14.

Feltham E (1991) Therapeutic touch and massage. Nursing Standard Vol 5 No 45.

Feifel H (1986) In Quest of the Spiritual Component for the Terminally Ill. Forward. Proceedings of Colloquin at York University.

Foreman EJ (1991) Planning Disaster Response Services: The Role of a Multi-Agency Steering Group. British Journal of Guidance & Counselling Vol 19 No 1.

Foss BM (1961) Determinants of Infant Behaviour Vol I. Methuen, London.

Foss BM (1963) Determinants of Infant Behaviour Vol II. Methuen, London.

Foss BM (1975) New Horizons in Psychology. Penguin, London.

Freidson E (1975) Dilemmas in the Doctor/Patient Relationship. In Cox C, Mead A, (Eds) A Sociology of Medical Practice. Op Cit p 285.

Frankl V (1963) Man's Search for Meaning (An Introduction to Logotherapy). NY Pocket Books, New York.

Fromer MJ (1981) Ethical Issues in Healthcare. CV Mosby, St Louis.

Fynne (1974) Mr God – This is Anna. Fontana, London.

Gibson M (1991) Order from Chaos: Responding to Traumatic Events. Venture Press.

Glik DC (1990) The Re-definition of the Situation: The Social Construction of Spiritual Healing Experiences. Soc. of Health and Illness Vol 12 No 2:151–168.

Goffman E (1968) Stigma (Chapter 1). Penguin, London.

Gorer G (1965) Death, Grief & Mourning in Contemporary Britain. Cresser, London.

Green J (1989 Death with Dignity. Nursing Times publication.

Hall J (1982) Dying and Bereavement. In Carr, AT, Psychology for Nurses and Health Visitors. British Psychological Society, MacMillan Press, London.

Harrison NJ (1993) Spirituality and Nursing Practice. Journal Clinical Nursing 2:211–217.

Hedley J (1988) Psychological Needs of Severely Ill & Dying Patients. To Sjoquist K , Nursing Times 5.3.

Hingley P (1991) The Cost of Stress and the Benefits of Stress Management. Occasional Paper No5, NASS.

Hopper E (1991) Shattered Dreams. Nursing Standard Vol 6 No 4:20–21.

ICN (1973) Code of Nursing Ethics. International Council of Nurses, Genoa.

Jackson I (1992) Bereavement Follow-Up Service in Intensive Care. Intensive & Critical Care Nursing 8:3.

Johnston M *et al.* (1992) The Impact of Death on Fellow Hospice Patients. British Journal of Medical Psychology 65:67–72.

Kellner Pringle M (1975) The Needs of Children (Chapter 1). Hutchinson, London.

Kretch D *et al.* (1962) Individual in Society. McGraw–Hill New York.

Krieger D (1979) The Therapeutic Touch. Prentice Hall Press, New York.

Krieger S (1981) The Renaissance Nurse Foundation of Holistic Health Practices. Lippincott, Philadelphia.

Kubler–Ross E (1969) On Death & Dying. MacMillan, N Yorks.

Labun E (1988) Spiritual Care: an element in Nursing Planning. Journal of Advanced Nursing Vol 3: 314–320.

Lawton D (1970) Social Class, Language and Education. R & KP, London.

Le Bowitz J, Connington B (1990) The Alexander Technique. Souvenir Press, London.

Lewis E, Bryan E (1988) Management of Perinatal Loss of a Twin. BMJ 297: 1321–1323.

Lewis JS (1994) Religion and Health. Is there an Association? Is it valid? Is it casual? Soc Science & Medicine Vol 88 No 11: 1478–1482.

Males J et al. (1990) Spiritual needs of people with a mental handicap. Nursing Standard Vol 4 No 48: 35–37.

Maslow A (1970) Motivation & Personality 2nd Edition. Harper & Row, New York.

McGilloway, Myco Au (1985) Nursing & Spiritual Care. Harper & Row, New York.

McGlone M (1991) Healing the Spirit. Holistic Nursing Practice Vol 4 No 4.

McKinley B, Brooks N (1991) Post Traumatic Stress Disorder Explained. Nursing Standard Vol 5 No 19.

McMahon R et al. (1991) Nursing as Therapy. Chapman & Hall, London.

Moulder C (1990) Miscarriage, Womens' Experiences & Needs. Pandora, London.

Muetzel P (1988) Therapeutic Nursing. In Pearson A (Ed) Primary Nursing in the Burford & Oxford Nursing Development Units. Croom Helm, London.

NASS (1992) A Charter for Staff Support. NASS.

Neuberger J (1987) Caring for Dying People of Different Faiths. Sainsbury Series. Austen Cornish, London.

Nichols K, Jenkinson J (1991) Leading a Support Group. Chapman & Hall, London.

Nouwen HJ (1987) The Wounded Healer.

Oakley A et al. (1984) Miscarriage. Fontana, London.

Oldfield V (1992) A Healing Touch. Nursing Standard Vol 6 No 44.

Owen GM et al. (1989) A Study of the Marie Curie Community Nursing Service. Marie Curie Memorial Foundation, London.

Owen GM (1990) Support Networks in Health Care. Occasional Paper No 1, NASS.

Owen GM (1993) Taking the Strain – Stress, Coping and Support Mechanisms. NASS Literature Review (revised annually).

Parkes CM (1972) Bereavement Studies of Grief in Adult Life. International Universities Press, New York.

Parkes CM (1975) Bereavement Studies of Grief in Adult Life 2nd Edition. International Universities Press, New York.

Parkes CM (1991) Planning for the Aftermath. Journal of the Royal Society of Medicine Vol 84.

Parsons T (1951) The Social System. Routeledge, Kegan & Paul, London.

Paton D (1990) Assessing the Impact of Disasters on Helpers. Counselling & Psychology Quarterly Vol 3 No 2: 149–152.

Pediani R (1992) Preparing to Heal. Nursing Times Vol 88 No 27: 68–69.

Penson J (1991) Complementary Therapies in Palliative Care for people with Cancer. Arnold, London.

Peplau HE (19690 Professional Closeness Nursing Forum Vol 8 No 4: 342, 360.

Peplau HE (1988) Interpersonal Relations in Nursing. MacMillan, London.

Peppers LG, Knapp RJ (1980) Motherhood & Mourning. Praeger, New York.

Peterson EA (1987) How to Meet your Client's Spiritual Needs. Journal of Psychological Nursing Vol 25 No 5: 34–38.

Rankin–Box D (1988) Complementary Health Therapies. A Guide for Nursing & The Caring Professions. Croom Helm, London.

Raphael B (1985) The Anatomy of Bereavement. A Handbook for the Caring Professions. Hutchinson, London.

Reed PG (1987) Spirituality and Well Being in Terminally Ill Hospitalised Adults. Research in Nursing & Health Vol 10: 335–344.

Mud & Stars, Report of an Experience (19910 The Impact of A Hospice Working Party. Sobell House Publications, Oxford.

Richman JM (1987) Stress Reduction for Hospice Workers.

Rosenfeld LB A Support Group Model in Stress and Burnout among Providers. The Hayworth Press.

Rogers C (1967) On Becomin a Person. Constable, London.

Ross B (1975) New Perspectives in Child Development. Penguin, London.

Rowan J (1990) Spiritual Experiences in Counselling. British Journal of Guidance & Counselling Vol 18 No 3: 232–248.

Rubin JG (1990) Critical Incident Stress Debriefing: Helping the Helpers. Journal of Emergency Nursing Vol 16 No 4.

Rumbold G (1986) Ethics in Nursing Practice. Balliere Tindall, London.

Rushton CM (1992) Care Giver Suffering in Critical Care Nursing. Heart & Lung Vol 21 No 3: 303–306.

Rutter M (1972) Maternal Deprivation Reassessed. Penguin, London.

Sadler C (1992) A Good Death. Nursing Times Vol 88 No 31: 16–17.

SANDS (1991) Guidelines for Professionals. Miscarriage, Stillbirth & Neonatal Death. SANDS, London.

Saunders C (1965) Watch With Me. Nursing Times Vol 61 No 48.

Saunders C (1969) The moment of truth, care for the dying patient. In Pearson L (Ed) Death and Dying, Current issues in Treatment of the Dying Person. Cleveland Press of Case Western University.

Saylor DE (1991) Pastoral Care of the Rehabilitative Patient. Rehabilitation Nursing Vol 16 No 3: 138–140.

Simpson H (1992) A Support Line that Restores Confidence. Professional Nurse.

Sims S (1988) In Wilson–Barnett et al. (1988) Nursing Issues & Research in Terminal Care. Wiley, London.

Sims S (1988) The Significance of Touch in Palliative Care. Palliative Medicine 2: 58–61.

Skevington S (1984) Understanding Nurses. The Social Psychology of Nursing. Bath Press, Avon.

Socken KL, Carson VJ (1987) Responding to Spiritual Needs of the Chronically Ill. Nursing Clinic of North America. Vol 22 No 3:603–611.

Speck P (1978) Loss & Grief in Medicine. Balliere Tindal, London.

Spinks P, Bowering P (1990) Staff Support. Paediatric Nursing, March 1990.

Stepnick A (1992) Preventing Spiritual Distress in The Dying Child. Journal of Psychological Nursing Vol 30: 1.

Stevenson C (1992) Appropriate Therapies for Nurses to Practice. Nursing Standard Vol 6 No 52.

Stewart A et al. (1992) An unfinished Story: Helping people come to terms with miscarriage. Professional Nurse Vol 7 No 8:656–660.

Stoll RI (1979) Guidelines for Spiritual Assessment. American Journal of Nursing 9: 1574–1577.

Storr A (1981) The Integrity of the Personality. Penguin, London.

Stoter DJ (1989) The Church's Role in Major Disaster. Occasional Paper, Churches Council for Health & Healing, London.

Stoter DJ (1991a) Spiritual care. In Pension J & Fisher R (Eds) Palliative Care for People with Cancer. Arnold, London.

Stoter DJ (1991b) Creating a Caring Culture. NASS Occasional paper No 6.

Strauss AL, Glasser BG (1968) Patterns of Dying, Sociology of Medical Practice. In Cox C & Mead A (Eds) Op Cir p 247.

Thomas J (1990) Supporting Parents when their Baby Dies. Nursing Standard Vol 5 No 6.

Thomas J (1991) Dignified in Death. Nursing Times Vol 87 No 29: 60–67.

Thomas J (1992) Supporting Parents when a Baby Dies. Care of the Critically Ill Vol 8 No 4: 172–174.

Truugpa CR (1978) Acknowledging Death. In Fosshage & Olsen (Eds) Healing. Human Sciences Press, New York.

Tschudin V, Marks–Maran D (1992) Ethics, A Review for Nurses. Balliere Tindall, London.

UKCC (1992) Code of Professional Conduct for the Nurse, Midwife and Health Visitor, 3rd edition. UKCC, London.

Vanstone WH (1977) Love's Endeavour, Love's Expense. Darton, Longman & Todd, London.

Veness D (1990) Spirituality in Counselling: A View from the Other Side. British Journal of Guidance & Counselling Vol 18 No 3: 250–260.

Wald FS (Ed) (1986) In Quest of the Spiritual Component of Care for the Terminally Ill. Feifel H (Foreword). Proceedings of a Colloquium. Yale University Press.

Wildwood C (1991) Aromatherapy. Element Books, London.

Winacott DW (1964) The Child, The Family & The Outside World. Penguin, London.

Woodruffe (1989) When Disaster Strikes: Staff Support after Major Incidents. Professional Nurse, June 1989.

Worden JW (1983) Grief Counselling & Grief Therapy. Tavistock Publications, London.

Wright B (1991) Sudden Death: Intervention Skills for the Caring Professions. Churchill Livingstone, Edinburgh.

INDEX

A

ABORTION 129
ACCEPTANCE
of other 20
ACCIDENT AND EMERGENCY
care in 95
needs in 91
trauma in 95
AFTER CARE 100
AIDS
social attitudes to 108
spiritual care in 107–8
**ALTERNATIVE THERAPIES/
MEDICINE**
acupuncture 48–9
aromatherapy 48–9
complimentary therapies 84
holistic care (See Holistic)
homeopathy 48
reflexology 48
relaxation 48
selection of 155
ANSWERS 15
integrated 154–5
to healing & care 154
ASSESSMENT
framework for 37–8
in spiritual need 43
of pain 60
or resources 45
recording 43
silence 41
touch 41–2
use of eyes 38
ATTITUDES
cultural 9
religious 9
spiritual 9
AWARENESS
personal 18–19
self 149

B

BELIEFS 10, 51
and practices 115–16
personal 10, 51, 120
religious 116–17
BEREAVEMENT
centre for 92
child's death 94
in miscarriage/still birth 93–94
loss in 61
response to 93
skills in care 87
spiritual care in 89
sudden death 96

C

CARE
critical 123
curative 123
delivery of 25

palliative 123
quality of 156
religious (see Religious)
spiritual (see Spiritual)
shared 45
terminal 123
total 11
5 Cs of 130
CARER(S) 9, 18–23
answers 28
anxieties for 28
care for 145–52
journey 11–12
professional 18, 27
resources (see Resources)
role 36
support for 28
CARING RELATIONSHIP 18,
22–23, 29
CHALLENGE(S)
chaplaincy 118–19
for carer 27
of caring 15
CHOICE(S) 48
in decision making 124–26
what are they? 129–30
CLIENT
centred 9
CODE
of ethics 124–29
of nursing practice 125–26
of professional practice 128
COMMUNICATION SKILLS 25,
31–6
answering 33
eye contact 32, 38–9
language 31–2
message 31
observation 32
process of 31
questioning 32–3
recipient 31
source 31
touch 32, 40–1
verbal 31
CONFIDENTIALITY 130
management of care 136
in team care 138
CONSUMER
participation 22
CONTROL
loss of 65
in alternative therapies 85–6
need for 85
CRITERIA
choices of 124–5
CULTURAL
background 21
CULTURE
attitudes 9–10
environmental 15
spiritual 15

CURE
nature of 154–5

D

DEATH
approach to 56–7
facing 104
fear of 14
of child 71–4
of parent 69–70
of spouse 70–1
patients response to impending 82
DECISIONS
between anvera 124
informed 124, 129–30
DEPRESSIVE DISORDERS 112–13
DILEMMAS 124–8
choices in 124
factors involved 125–6
limited resources 126
DISEASE 154
DYING
approach to 56–7
models of 56–7
personal experience 57
phases of 56–7
fears of 14

E

ENCOUNTER 39
ETHICAL PRINCIPLES 124–6
codes 126–8
on core of spiritual care 129–30
relevant to spiritual care 127–8
EUTHANASIA 129
EXPECTATIONS
in different roles 56
of pain 60
of recovery/cure 82–3
EXPLORATION
into spiritual care 119

F

FAITH
multi-faith society 117
variations in 117
FAMILY
as a resource 63
effects on (of loss) 73
influences 4, 10, 19, 20
life 4
resources for 139
support for 141
FEAR(S) 27
of death 14
FEELINGS 35
child's 75
emotions related to illness 75
guilt, anger etc. 73
in grief 61
of anger 35
of pain 35

of rejection 35
strong emotions 72

H
HABIT
loss of 65, 68
powerful element 65, 68
HEALING
approach(es) to 154–5
nature of 89, 154–5
response to 81
through alternative therapy 84
HOLISTIC
care 2, 48

I
ILLNESS
long term 102–7
terminal 103–5
nature of 154
INFLUENCES
environmental 19
family 4, 10, 19–20
from parents 10
INTENSIVE CARE
needs in 96
provision of care 96
IN-VITRO FERTILISATION 126

J
JOURNEY 4
Of life 8, 11–14
Together 11–14
Carers' 12

K
KNOWLEDGE 117

L
LIFE
meaning of 127
preservation 131
quality of 127
LISTENING
in communication 31
skills of 34–6
to family 103–4
LOSS
bereavement 62
of a child 63
of body image 64
of control 65
of communication 65
of habit 65, 68
of parent(s) 69–70
of a spouse 70–1
of self image 64
potential 63–4, 71
related to childbirth 75
sudden 62

M
MAJOR DISASTERS
informal debriefing 98
spiritual care in 97
support in 96
MENTAL HEALTH

spiritual care for 111
MENTAL ILLNESS 111
MISCARRIAGE
loss in 74–5
MODELS 38
Bradshaw's Taxonomy 6
Maslow's Hierachy 3
MORAL
dilemmas 124
principles 124
values 124, 127

N
NEED(S) 1
expressed 6
felt 5
in unsuspected situations 91
recognition of 5–6
special 90–1
unmet 5
unspoken 6

O
OBSTETRICS
provision of care 93
special needs in 93

P
PAIN
as a response 59–67
anxiety & tension in 61
causes of 60
expectations of 61
expression of 35
factors influencing 60
of caring 147
of others 147
of suffering 59
PARTNERSHIP
relationship 22, 29
with family/friends 156
PATIENT('S)
centred 9
long-stay 102-5
name 25
need (see Needs)
participation 22
quality of care 145
response (see Response)
rights 28
PAEDIATRICS
provision of care 94–5
PERCEPTION
of person 40
skills of 40
PERSON
unique 37
PERSONAL
beliefs 21
experiences 21
skills 42
PERSONALITY
formation 19
secure 20
PERSPECTIVES
influences on 127–8
on decision making 127

PRACTICES
of faith 10
PREGNANCY
termination of 127, 129
PROVISION FOR
alcoholics/drug abuses 108
community care 106
HIV/AIDS patients 107–8
long term care 102–5
spiritual care in general 91, 102–5

Q
QUESTIONS 15
answering 33–4
asking 32–3
carers' 15
oblique 33
open 33
probe 33

R
RECOVERY
spiritual care during 109–11
REHABILITATION
spiritual care during 109
RELATIONSHIP(S) 3, 12
caring 8, 18–23
comfortable 25
establishing 24–7
helping 26
partnership in 79, 85
personal 9–10
secure 20
through life 9
RELATIVES
special care 99
RELIGION 7
RELIGIOUS
affiliation 4, 9
attitudes 9
blackmail 9
care 9–10
community 10
need(s) 120
practices 120–22
requirements 153
RESPONSE
& public persona 55
anxiety in 60
child's 75–6
emotional 57–8
factors influencing 58–65
internal 54
problem solving 57
potential loss to 63–71
of patient 53–87
of sibling's 73
of patient's to dying 77–8
nature of 56
to dying 56–7
to healing 81
to illness 62
to loss (see Loss)
to pain 60
to recovery 82–7
to suffering 59
sudden loss 59

to trauma 78
RIGHTS
individual 22
of individual 129, 131
patient 28
to discontinue 59
RESOURCES
assessment of 45
for patient and family 139
for spiritual care 139
in volunteers 140
team 47
RESOURCES OF CARER 19, 45–52
beliefs 47–8
knowledge 47–8
personal 18–45
personal gifts 46
professional 47–8
skills 46
staff support (see 'Staff Support')
RESPONSE 9–10
skills of 29
learned 35
RESPONSIBILITY(IES)
of managers 152
ROLES
and expectations 56
and relationships 134–6
of parents 71
professional 69
patient's 54
in the team 63
ROLES & RELATIONSHIPS
in spiritual care 119
in team work 136
in the caring team 134–6

S
SACRAMENT(AL)
ministry 10
SELF
development 19
knowledge 21
SILENCE
in assessment 41
SKILLS
of acquisition 31–6
of assessment 37–44
of carers 31–6
of communication 25, 31–6
of coping 35
of counselling 32
of interpreting 35
of practical 31–6
of response 29
of silence 32
skill mix 134
supportive 35
use of sense 40
SOCIALISATION 19
SPIRITUAL 2–3
approach to care 4–5
attitudes 9–10
behaviour 3
being 3
care 3–16, 28, 33
core of care 9

culture 9–10
dimension 2–3, 10
health 140–44
journey 11–14
long term needs 102
nature 3
need 2–7
person 19
rituals 3
SPIRITUALITY 2, 3, 6
SPIRITUAL CARE
core of 155
delivery of 134
demands of 148
during rehabilitation 109
factors affecting 119
for staff 145
for the elderly 103–4
for HIV/AIDS patients 107–8
for alcoholics/drug addicts 108
implications for 120
in community care 107
in multi-faith society 116–17
in terminal illness 105
integrating force 156
long term 105
– nature of 153
provision for 102
SPIRITUAL NEED
of staff 145–7
STAFF SUPPORT
from team 49–50
individual approach 147–8
in ICU 96
in major disasters 97
organisational approach 148
personal 50–1
support network 49
3 levels of 147
STIGMA 56
SUPPORT
for carers 25
for staff 35
SUPPORT GROUPS
as a resource 139
confidentiality 130
for carers 140
for family 103
for patients 103, 139,
for staff 143, 150
for bereavement 142
success of 151
value of 142–3

T
TEAM WORK 155
in spiritual care 136
pressures in 137
THEORIES & MODELS
death & dying 82
examples of 55, 62
use and abuse of 55
THREAT
of loss of control 35
of rejection 35
of unknown 13
TOUCH

conveying messages 42
healing agent 41
in communication 32, 39–40
skills of 41
therapeutic 49
TRUST
partnership in 156
TRUTH(S)
absolute 120
respect for 120
whole 120

V
VALUE(S) 4
judgements 5
of individual 156
VOLUNTEERS
for community care 106
role of 140
support for 140
training for 140
use of 140

W
WHOLENESS
concept of 154
in spiritual care 153
of mind & body 154, 156